Safe
and
Sound

The Complete Guide
to First Aid and
Emergency Treatment
for Children and Young
Adults

Linda Wolfe

Medical Editor: Dr David Zideman

Foreword by Esther Rantzen
Illustrations by Gordon Munro and Branwen Thomas

Hodder & Stoughton
LONDON SYDNEY AUCKLAND

British Library Cataloguing in Publication Data
Wolfe, Linda
    Safe and Sound: Complete Guide to First
    Aid and Emergency Treatment for Children and Young Adults
    I. Title
    616.02

ISBN 0-340-56996-4

First published in Great Britain 1993
Illustrations © Gordon Munro 1993
Illustrations © Branwen Thomas 1993

Every care has been taken on the advice given in this book on First Aid. This
advice has been taken in consultation with St John Ambulance and leading medical
authorities. The author or publishers cannot, however, take any responsibility for
any loss or damage suffered as a result of any errors or omissions in the advice
given or in the text.

Published by Hodder and Stoughton,
a division of Hodder and Stoughton Ltd,
Mill Road, Dunton Green, Sevenoaks, Kent TN13 2YA
Editorial Office: 47 Bedford Square, London WC1B 3DP

Front cover logo by Signal Communications Ltd
Photoset in Plantin by SX Composing Ltd, Rayleigh, Essex
Printed in Great Britain by BPCC Hazells Ltd, Aylesbury, Bucks,
Member of BPCC.

ACKNOWLEDGEMENTS

I would like to thank the following people and organisations for helping me compile the information for *Safe and Sound*:

Terrence Bate (Assistant Chief Veterinary Officer, RSPCA), Maddie Blackburn (Research Fellow ASBAH UK), Tony Brett-Young (Communications Officer, National Playing Fields Association), British Epilepsy Association, Steve Crone and Fiona McLean (National Asthma Campaign), Maggie Dodgson (Child Abuse Police Worker), Eating Disorders Association, Paul Farmer (Press Officer, Samaritans), Iona Fisher (Media Council), Martin Flaherty (Press Officer, London Ambulance Service), Geoffrey Green and Kate Thomas (Foundation for the Study of Infant Deaths), Ruth Grigg and Melissa Dear (Family Planning Association), Dr John I. Harper (Consultant Paediatric Dermatologist, Senior Lecturer, Institute of Child Health, Great Ormond Street Hospital), Derek Hirst (Research/Information, ROSPA), Graham Hood (Head of the Youth Department, British Diabetic Association), Andy Horne (Director, Westminster Drugs Project), Fredwyn Hosier (Director of Barnet, Enfield and Haringey Samaritans), Dr Margaret Jones (Brook Advisory Service), Divisional Officer Malcolm Kelly (London Fire Brigade), Helen Kenwood (Child Abuse Social Worker), Catherine Lyons (Senior Nurse Manager, Hammersmith Hospital), Margaret McGowan (The National Children's Play and Recreation Unit), Rosemary Morle (SCODA the Standing Conference on Drug Abuse), Dr K.G. Nicholson (Consultant in Infectious Diseases [Rabies]), Louise Pankhurst and Dr Sara Levene (Child Accident Prevention Trust), Malcolm Parsons (Press Officer, British Railways Board), Catharine Pointer (Librarian, The Compassionate Friends), Powerbreaker (thanks for RCD photo), Press Office of the London Ambulance Headquarters, Helen Reilly (*General Practitioner* magazine), Safety Research Unit (Consumer Safety – Department of Trade and Industry), Tom Sanders (Water Safety at ROSPA), Mr A. Sharif (Consultant Orthopaedic Surgeon), Pauline Shelley (Action for Sick Children [NAWCH]), David Smith (Dave's Disc Doctor Service), Sylvia Tadd and Richard Green (Managers at the NSPCC Child Protection Helpline), Julian Turner (Off-Centre), Ian Wardle (Lifeline), Dr Nolan Wengrowe GP, and the staff at the Heathfielde Medical Centre.

The author and publishers gratefully acknowledge the kind permission of Michele Elliott to reproduce her codes for Kidscape from *Keeping Safe: A Practical Guide to Talking with Children*.

The medical photographs and X-rays are courtesy of the Hospital for Sick Children, the Westminster Hospital and Guy's Hospital, with special thanks to all the medical library staff for their help and assistance.

The illustrations of how to remove fish hooks (page 212) are by courtesy of *The General Practitioner*, 13 December 1991; 17 January 1992; and the toxic substance symbols (page 227) by courtesy of the British Safety Council.

I would like to thank the following people for their special contribution or support:

Tim Binding, Dr Brien Cooke (Consultant in Public Health Medicine, Health Education Authority), Professor Alan Craft (Consultant Paediatrician, Royal Victoria Infirmary, Newcastle), Kathryn Dymoke and Mark Le Fanu (Society of Authors), Sue Griffin (Training Officer of the National Childminders' Association), Lt. Commander John Hammond (St John Ambulance Association and Brigade), Malcolm Keene (Consultant ENT Surgeon, St Bartholomew's Hospital), Ros Meek (Health Visitors Association), Maureen O'Hagan (Manager of the Council for Early Years Award), Miss Winifrid Joan Robson (Consultant Paediatrician in Accident and Emergency at Alder Hey Children's Hospital, Liverpool and Director of the Rainbow Centre, Liverpool, for abused children), Jenny Rogers! Professor Jo Sibert (Consultant Paediatrician, Llandough Hospital, Cardiff and Trustee of the Child Accident Prevention Trust), Nicola Solomon (Stephens Innocent), Lynne Walsh (Head of Press Office), Lucy Thorpe (both of the Health Education Authority) and Bob Watkins (photographer).

A special message to Arthur Ward of Signal Communications, Graphics Designer of the logo for *Safe and Sound*. You are the best, Arthur. *Please get well soon*.

I would like to extend my grateful thanks to those people who have worked directly with me on the book and its complexities:

Jayne Booth – for slowly but inexorably pulling me out of the mire and for your humour, delightful sensitivity and seeming indefatigability whilst you were doing it.

Celia Levett – for all your painstaking work.

David Zideman – for your wonderful guidance, support and sheer breadth of knowledge. Your incisive comments and ruthless editing have hopefully helped many parents to keep their children even more *Safe and Sound* than if I had written it without you!

Jon Roseman – for all the energy, enthusiasm and support. Lovely!

Gordon Munro and Branwen Thomas – for your special contribution. The beautiful illustrations that you have created between you have really helped to clarify what I was trying to say in the text.

And lastly my special thanks to Esther Rantzen for finding the time (from where?) to write the foreword. My love to you.

CONTENTS

To David, who keeps me safe and sound.

To Kate (especially Kate), Oliver and Betsy, without whom this book would not have been written!

And to Ella and Hazel for staying cool.

Thank you for your love, patience and support and for putting up with me through all the angst!

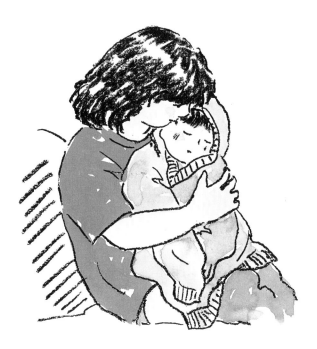

If you have saved a child's life as a result of using this book, please let us know so that we can update our research for the next edition.

FOREWORD

Nobody can predict exactly when they are going to need the valuable advice and protection contained in this book. I know from my own life and from the many letters I receive how crucial it is to know exactly how to cope when disaster strikes.

When the baby rolls off the sofa, you need to act swiftly and effectively. When a toddler swallows a penny, and begins to choke, you have three minutes to pat her on the back and resuscitate her. Just reading this book prepares you in advance to act rather than panic, and of course consulting the book in an emergency will enable you also to seek appropriate professional help if you need it.

I think this will become a secular family bible on the shelf constantly dipped into, well-thumbed, of particular use in the life and death moments that strike the best organised families out of the blue. I only wish it had been around the night my baby rolled off the sofa, and the day my husband set fire to his legs. It would have saved us desperate seconds of indecision and anxiety, and given us the confidence to do the right thing, the right way, to make sure the least damage was done.

Esther Rantzen

INTRODUCTION

One evening when my daughter Kate was one, she became very ill. As a nurse I knew how ill she was but, as I was calling the doctor, her heart and breathing stopped. What I didn't expect was the horror and sheer panic I felt when I realised I would have to breathe for her and restart her heart with my fingertips if I was to save her life. The panic blotted out what I was trying to do and if David, my husband, hadn't been standing behind me saying, 'Gently, she's only a baby,' I might have forgotten the difference between saving an adult's life and saving a child's.

Often parents and carers don't know what to do when an accident happens or a child becomes seriously ill. Perhaps the idea of a situation where your child's life is in danger is too horrific to think about and the only way for you to deal with it is to say, 'It *couldn't* happen to my child.' But many lives could be saved if the first person on the scene – usually a parent, but often the child-minder, au pair, grandparent or babysitter – knew what to do. After all, ANY first aid given to the child is better than none.

It is vital, therefore, for those caring for children to learn what to do. Children have many more accidents and become very ill more quickly than adults but it is amazing how few parents and carers feel confident to deal with an emergency.

There is nothing I can write, however, that can take the place of a real, live First Aid Course. You may have bought this book instead of doing a course, but 'as well as' would give you much more confidence. There are some things that you just cannot learn from a book so if you really want to crack first aid, treat yourself to a St John Ambulance First Aid Course. It is hard work but the standard of the teaching is excellent and at the end of the course you really feel you could cope with any emergency (see page 16). If going on a course is not possible for you for the time being, then this book will give you the 'basics' and will be a constant source of vital information.

Accidents tend to happen when parents are under stress. It's not because we don't care but because we're thinking about other things. Surprise, surprise! Working mothers and fathers are under an enormous strain and any parent will tell you how difficult it is to run a home, organise the kids and put in a full, part-time or job-share working day. But even those at home all day with a number of children cannot keep an eye on all of them all the time (see Chapter 32 on Preventing Accidents).

This book will help you to react quickly and calmly when accidents happen so that you can always be prepared for an emergency situation.

What happens when a child has an accident

The bad news is that children have more accidents than adults and the *effect* of the accident is more harmful. This is because the impact on their little bodies is greater as they are so much more fragile.

The good news is that, given the right treatment, a child's healing power is far greater than an adult's, and they tend to bounce back with amazing speed even after the most appalling injuries. Notice how much more quickly a toddler's wound heals compared to that of her grandparents, for example, or even her parents.

To understand what happens when a child has an accident or is ill, it helps to know how the body works. In Chapter 2 on How the Body Works you will find illustrations of the body, its organs, bones and the blood system. Although you will already have a rough idea of where everything goes, this is to remind you, so that IF your child is injured you will feel more confident to deal with it.

It's frightening sometimes to think of where we leave our children: kindergartens and schools are usually all right (although individual teachers and child-minders don't *have* to hold an up-to-date First Aid Certificate); but Cubs and Brownies, sports centres and holiday schemes *must be checked* to make sure that someone on the staff has first aid training.

Interestingly, parents often feel uncomfortable about approaching organisers to ask if they have had first aid training. I'm not quite sure why this is. We are basically talking about our children's lives and parents should always ask if those in charge feel confident to deal with emergency situations before leaving children with anyone they don't know.

Most accidents to children, however, happen in the 'safety' of the home. Children are very curious and want to find out how things work. It's not just being naughty when they tip out a drawer or want to see what is in that lovely, shiny, bubbling pan.

One day, squat down to child level and try to see things from their position. Look at trailing kettle flexes (the cause of the most horrific scalding accidents) and shiny pan handles sticking over the cooker top; look again at boxes of matches and plug sockets; peer inside cupboards full of different coloured and shaped bottles of bleach and disinfectants, cleaners and liquids that will burn. It may sound daft, but it might help you understand how different things are from a child's eye view.

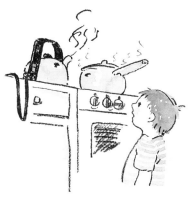

Looking at things from a child's eye view.

In *Safe and Sound* I have looked at some of the commonest childhood accidents and illnesses as well as those that probably will never happen to your child but which you should be aware of; Chapter 32 on Preventing Accidents was written under the eye of Professor Jo Sibert, who apart from being a paediatrician is also a trustee of the Child Accident Prevention Trust.

The idea of this book is not to send you scatty with worry but to help you wise up and open your eyes to what could happen to your child and

11

then to show you how to deal with it.

The difference between this book and other general books on first aid is that *Safe and Sound* is for PARENTS. I have tried to think through what parents *would* do, rather than what they *should* do if their child were ill or injured. My belief is that no matter how stupid it may be, in some circumstances a parent would jump in the water to save a drowning child *in spite of* putting herself or himself in enormous danger, and *in spite of* not being able to swim (see Chapter 13 on Drowning). If a child has set herself alight, a parent would probably risk burning herself or himself to save the child's life (see Chapter 7 on Burns and Scalds). *Safe and Sound* is also about keeping parents and other carers safe while getting a child out of a dangerous situation.

One of the most important things to remember is that for a child to have his mother's arms around him when he is ill or injured is 75 per cent of healing. Don't ever forget how important you are to that process and that if you do nothing else but hold and comfort your child and learn the basics from this book he will be safe and sound.

When a child has a serious accident you need to have your wits about you. If the child is conscious, always, *always* reassure her – a warm, soothing and, hopefully, familiar voice can be the first step towards recovery.

Try not to tell your child off no matter how stupid she has been or how dangerous her behaviour. It isn't going to help at this stage. This is much easier said than done: your first reaction may be to scream at her that she could have killed herself.

When you feel you have done all you can in the way of first aid and the ambulance is on its way, try to grab the child's favourite teddy or toy, to take with her. Cuddling is comforting but she may be too badly injured for you to cuddle her.

In a bad accident it is often difficult to know what to do first. For instance, when a child is severely injured it's no good racing around getting bandages to stop the bleeding of a badly gashed leg if at the other end she has stopped breathing.

HOW TO USE THIS BOOK

It would be useful to read *Safe and Sound* whenever you have the time and space to take in the background information. Do not wait until an accident happens; in an emergency it will be impossible to do this.

● The chapters are arranged alphabetically and I have included in each chapter a description of the injury or illness, what to look for and what to do.

● In each chapter, I have taken the main points of the immediate things to do to save a child's life – or in the case of the non-emergency chapters, to make her more comfortable – and put them on one page. This is called the Emergency Page.

● The book is bound in such a way that when you open it, in an emergency, *the page should stay open at the place you need.*

● I have tried to avoid using too many medical terms in the book but there will be things doctors say which you might not understand and which you may feel uncomfortable asking about; you can look these up in the various sections or you can track them down in the index (page 288).

● As you will see, I have referred to your child as 'she' in some chapters and 'he' in others. I have referred to everyone as 'children' even though some may be teenagers. Some information is more about boys than girls – and vice versa. For clarity, so as not to mix them up with the child, I have called doctors and dentists 'he' and nurses and health visitors 'she'. I am bound to have offended someone but I have tried not to!

I can only hope that you never have to use the advice in this book, but being familiar with it will give you more confidence to keep your child safe.

1 PREPARATION AND PRACTICAL ISSUES

Every child will have an accident of some kind before he or she is fifteen, so it is always sensible to be prepared.

Before we begin the basic principles of first aid, however, it is worth thinking about all the practical issues that surround a child who has had an accident or who has become ill.

For instance, if you have to ask a neighbour or relative to call the ambulance in an emergency, will he or she have all the information they need?

Is your telephone number (including the area code) printed on the handset? The new phones often don't have this and while you may know your own number, the neighbour who has dashed in to help may not. This is the first thing the emergency operator will ask for. (It is possible, even for you, to forget your own telephone number in an emergency.)

Make a typewritten (or clearly handwritten) emergency list of the following, perhaps in the front of the household telephone book:

● Your DOCTOR'S name and telephone number, and the emergency number so that if it is before or after surgery hours you know where to get hold of him.

● The work telephone number of your WIFE/HUSBAND/PARTNER and where else they can be contacted in an emergency, for example through the foreman, manager, portable telephone, pager, and so on.

● The numbers of two NEIGHBOURS OR RELATIVES you can trust. You need to think through who would look after the other children in an emergency if you had to take an ill or injured child to hospital.

● The LOCAL HOSPITAL can come in very useful. In an emergency, if your GP is not contactable for a considerable time (perhaps it's the middle of the night) and you need urgent advice but you don't feel you need to call for an ambulance, the hospital Accident and Emergency Sister will sometimes be able to help. I don't recommend you to do this on a regular basis, but on the two occasions (in eight years) I have rung, they have been extremely helpful.

● Finally, if at all possible, leave a telephone number with the babysitter, wherever you are going. Two or three hours is a long time in a small child's life and anything can happen. You will feel a lot happier if you are at the end of a phone.

It is important, once the children are old enough, to teach them how to contact the emergency services. It could be extremely useful, for instance if for any reason the children find themselves alone in the house. It is not unknown for the babysitter, au pair or nanny to get an unexpected attack of the blues and decide to pack her bags and go, no matter how many children she has to look after or how old they are. Or if they are being looked after by the babysitter, who could be the sixteen-year-old next door – she may not know the emergency procedures. It can only be comforting to you that your five-, six- or seven-year-old could summon help if she had to. It is also useful to talk to the children about this occasionally and to play 'what if' so that in an emergency they are semi-prepared. (You don't have to play it every day!)

Something may also happen to you and you may need to rely on your child in an emergency.

CALLING THE AMBULANCE

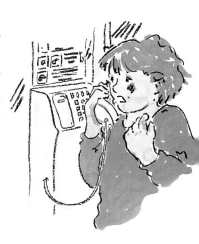

WHEN YOU DIAL 999 remember you will be put through to the *emergency operator* and *not* direct to the Ambulance Service. At this point you will be asked, 'What service do you require?' (Fire, Police or Ambulance) and, 'What is your number?' (the number from which you are dialling, so that if for any reason the call gets interrupted, they can ring you back right away). You may not be able to get through immediately to the Ambulance Service and in an emergency every second can seem like hours. *Very* occasionally you may even get a recorded message. DO NOT HANG UP. British Telecom has not let go of your call. If you feel you must see to your child's injuries, *leave the phone off the hook* and come back to the phone as soon as you can.

WHEN YOU GET THROUGH TO THE AMBULANCE be prepared to tell the operator:

1   *Exactly* where you are. You may not be at home. Give as accurate a description as possible as Ambulance Central Control may not know your area. Remember, if you are using a phone box there is a notice on the inside wall, giving the address. If that is missing, look for a landmark you think the ambulance driver would recognise and *remember to give directions as to where they'll find the injured child*.

2   Give the telephone number, if possible. Not all handsets have the number attached.

3   Describe the type of accident, for example a child has fallen through a glass door.

4   Tell them what has happened, for example large cuts on hands, face and leg. Bleeding badly.

5   Say what you have done so far, such as: 'I have put pressure on the

15

wound to stop the bleeding and raised the limbs, but the child has lost a lot of blood and is in a bad state of shock.' If you don't know what to do, say so.

6   They need as much detail as possible about your child's condition and what you think has happened *before they arrive*, so that they can be ready to give the appropriate emergency treatment when they reach the child.

7   If the child is seriously injured or is dangerously ill, the ambulance operator may give advice over the telephone while the ambulance is on its way to you.

ALWAYS REMEMBER: *let the operator put the telephone down first* in case there is something else she wants to ask you. It is all too easy, in a panic, to gabble the details and slam the phone down, forgetting to give the address of where the child is lying injured.

Be aware of how to attract attention. This is no time to think of the neighbours – shouting out of an open window is one way if you think the ambulance won't find you easily. If it's dark, tell the operator you'll try to turn the lights off and on in the front room; but see if you can get someone to do this for you.

If you are on your own, turn on all the lights in the front rooms of the flat or house and open the curtains. The main thing is that the ambulance should find you as quickly as possible. If you live in a block of flats and feel it may be difficult to find you, try and get someone to stand at the corner of your block to direct the ambulance.

A word of warning. The Ambulance Service told me of a case where someone was waiting outside a house to direct the driver to a patient. The ambulance came speeding along the road and the man stepped in front of it to prevent it, as he thought, from going straight past. The ambulance couldn't stop in time and ran him over. It wasn't going to that house but was answering a call a few streets away.

Just to remind you

NOTHING can take the place of a First Aid Course. St John Ambulance hopes to start a special course for parents, child-minders and carers. All St John First Aid Courses are hard work, extremely thorough and great fun. You come out feeling more confident and much more able to deal with any of the minor or major injuries that may happen to a child in your care. If you are interested you can get details from your local phone book or contact:

St John Ambulance Association and Brigade
1 Grosvenor Crescent, London SW1X 7EF.
Tel. 071 235 5231

TAKING A CHILD TO HOSPITAL

About three million children are admitted to Accident and Emergency hospitals (A & E) every year. In inner city areas, one child in five is seen in A & E after having an accident or a serious illness. For many of these children it is their first experience of hospital.

Everyone gets frightened by illness and pain, especially if it is sudden and caused by an accident, but many Accident and Emergency departments are more geared to the needs of adults than to children.

Children admitted to hospitals in an emergency should be seen *separately* in A & E by doctors and nurses used to dealing with children. The Department of Health recommended this twenty years ago but many hospitals still have not followed the recommendations.

This is what should happen once a child arrives in hospital. She should be seen in a separate waiting area with a specially trained nurse to welcome her into the department. Hammersmith Hospital in London has a side room attached to their A & E department where the child can be examined quietly and calmly while her parents stay nearby. They are well away from the eyes of other adults and they feel much safer.

If your child has an accident or is suddenly taken ill and you have to call for an ambulance try to think through how you are going to manage and what you need to do before you go to the hospital.

Are you on your own and is there someone to look after the other children? Quickly make a list, or tell someone who can pick them up where the children are. Tell them to let your partner or a friend know what has happened.

You may find yourself on your own with the other children and no one there to help. In that case take them all with you in the ambulance to the hospital; this is not ideal but you may have no choice.

Make sure your child is lying 'comfortably' (as much as possible anyway) in the Recovery Position, or whatever position you have put her in to keep her safe. It may be impossible to leave her for a second but, if you can, try to collect a few things that she or you might need. What comes to mind are her own belongings to make the child feel more secure in unfamiliar surroundings:

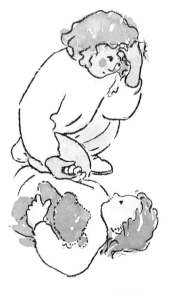

- If your child has a teddy or 'comforter' take it with you no matter how scruffy it is and even if she has grown out of it. Ill children often go back a few years emotionally – something you should bear in mind if she suddenly starts wetting the bed again, or wants to go back from cup to bottle.

- If she has a dummy or bottle take that as well, even if she rarely uses it. She might like to in hospital.

17

● She may already be in her pyjamas or nightgown, but if she isn't, and if you have time to find them, take her favourite pair. It is not a good idea to put a child in 'strange' clothes, which may really upset an already frightened child.

● These are the most important things for a small child; but even an older child might not object to a much-loved old teddy being packed with her 'Walkman'.

● Don't forget her wash-bag – any child from the age of about five appreciates her own wash things.

Remember, depending on the sort of accident, the child may feel she is being punished by being sent to hospital, particularly if she has to stay overnight. You may have to work hard to reassure her that you are not angry with her and that it is not her fault. Even if she did behave stupidly, now isn't the time to tell her. Tell her she is coming home as soon as she is better.

She needs to know too how much you love her; it is at times like this that she needs telling again. This may sound over the top, but sick children get most peculiar ideas in their heads and they need to be reassured that everything is all right.

As far as your own needs are concerned, it will depend on how much time you have got before you leave. If you can manage it, take some of the following: tea-bags, nightwear (or you might be happy to bed down in a track-suit, for instance), wash-bag and any make-up things you need to make you feel more human (if you are not getting much sleep), a book or something for you to do – the day can seem very long, especially if the child is sleeping.

Hospital parents' rooms usually have a kettle and somewhere to sit, but not always tea-bags. Some have everything you could want if you moved in for a long stay, but others have nothing.

She may not want you to leave, and you are helping her get better by being there; but it doesn't mean that you have to be bored – no matter how much you love her!

If your child has attacks of some kind on a regular basis, each time having to go to hospital for a night or more, it is a good idea to pack a bag in readiness (a plastic carrier bag is excellent), with the bits and pieces that can make the time pass more pleasantly. You can then add the last-minute items as you go through the door.

Alternatively if you think she might have to stay in hospital because of her injuries or illness, then it might be a good idea to pack some things anyway – you can always bring them home again. If you don't have time before you go, you might want to make a list of things for your partner or friend to bring, when he or she comes in.

When the ambulance arrives

Most ambulance men and women are really understanding and they will quickly give your child the appropriate emergency treatment she needs. If at all possible give as much detail as you can about her condition to the emergency switchboard – then the ambulance crew will know exactly what to do the moment they see your child. Otherwise they have to start finding out what has happened once they arrive and may waste precious moments.

Many ambulances now have Paramedics on board. These people have had special experience and training over and above their ambulance training.

If your child is very badly injured and the ambulance officers and Paramedics have to do some tricky emergency treatment, they may need a lot of room to manoeuvre in the ambulance. There may be things going on which look extremely alarming. If they have time to explain they will (they definitely will if they have children of their own), otherwise trust that what they are doing is the *least amount* of emergency treatment that they have to do, to get her safely to hospital.

Ambulance officers do not give drugs generally except oxygen, Paramedics on the other hand do. They have strict guidelines, however, about what drugs they may give and *how* they are given. The two main ways are by injection either under the skin or through a 'drip' into the vein. They can also give drugs for the child to breathe in through a mask (nebuliser), for instance in bad asthmatic attacks (see Chapter 5 on Asthma).

They may suggest that your partner or friend follows separately – either by private car, taxi or public transport. Obviously in a grave emergency the ambulance has its blue light flashing and neither car nor taxi could (or should try to) keep up. However, normally they will encourage both of you to go in the ambulance with your child.

Once in the ambulance

Try not to panic – no matter what they are trying to do to help her. These people are very skilled and if they can save her, they will. You may have been wonderfully calm up to this point but when the full horror of the situation hits you, you may suddenly want to 'throw a wobbly'. Don't do this yet, there will be plenty of time later.

Your child needs you to be calm, strong and reassuring – although you probably need a parent to hold your hand right now! Just keep talking quietly to her, no matter what's going on, until you get to the hospital.

Once you get to hospital

The staff are usually sympathetic – try not to panic or fuss and let them do their job. However, once the emergency is over, your child may have to stay in hospital for all sorts of reasons.

If it is at all possible you will want to stay with her although you may

19

not be able to if you have other children at home. The days when parents were discouraged from staying with their child in hospital are over, thank goodness, but don't expect a suite at the Ritz – the 'provisions' are pretty basic. Most times you will get a camp bed to put up next to your child's and even some blankets and sheets! Occasionally if the nursing staff are very busy, you may just get a chair or a blanket on the floor. But if your child is very poorly you won't mind that and you will probably just be grateful that you can be with her.

Most nurses welcome parents to the ward and feel that they have a valuable contribution to make to the child's recovery and want to involve them in her overall nursing care. However, occasionally you may find a nurse who is not so enthusiastic (she may have had a bad experience with some over-anxious mother and she may feel that parents just spell stress).

There may be a situation when *you* may not want to stay with your child, particularly if the medical staff have something unpleasant to do to her and you feel you cannot cope with seeing your child so miserable or in pain. (You may also have other children at home whom you are feeling guilty about.) Try to talk to the nurse looking after your child and explain how you feel. She will understand and encourage you to come back as soon as you feel able.

It is important that once your child has been admitted to the ward you have a word with the nurse planning her care so you can talk about how the accident happened or when the child first became ill, and discuss the special needs of your child – what she calls things for instance, especially the toilet. There is nothing worse for a nurse looking after a sick child who wants, or needs, some simple thing that would make her less anxious or more comfortable when no one understands what she is saying.

You might want to talk to the nurse about you and your family circumstances – such as other little ones at home (there may be all sorts of horrendous things going on for you that you might want her to know about or *not*, but she is not a mind-reader and it might help you if you shared your problems).

You should feel free to do all the things you think your child wants to make her feel more comfortable – the nurses will soon tell you if you are in the way. They will really appreciate your help, as long as you are not over-fussy and they are allowed to get on with their job, which is to make your child better.

Don't be afraid to ask to see the doctor and to find out exactly what is the matter with your child, how long she is expected to stay in hospital and so on. If the nurse in charge says that the doctor is too busy to see anyone, you must be strong enough to ask when he will be free. If you feel it is urgent, then say so, quietly and clearly; otherwise agree to make an appointment for as soon as possible. Then ask, at 'fair' intervals, if the nurse has managed to contact him. Make a list of things you want to ask – it's much easier to remember if you have them written down.

Believe it or not, some doctors are sometimes a little afraid of parents. They don't get any special training in dealing with them, so they often don't know what to say! So no matter how anxious you are about your child, go easy on the doctor. I don't mean don't ask him straight questions and expect straight answers, but don't necessarily expect the 'bedside manner' – it sometimes happens, but not always. This doesn't mean he isn't a good doctor, only that he isn't good at talking about it. (Having said that, some doctors are absolutely lovely – often because they have children themselves.)

During her stay in hospital your child may see lots of different doctors, while the nurses should stay roughly the same, although they change at night and on 'days off'. After she has been seen by the Accident and Emergency doctor there are three main *types* of doctor she might see:

- The paediatricians look after the general *medical* welfare of your child. They have a special training just to look after children.

- Then there are the surgeons (they are called Mr, Mrs or Miss rather than 'Doctor'). These are the doctors who perform any operation the child needs, either through injury or illness.

- Lastly there are the anaesthetists. These are the special doctors who will give your child a general anaesthetic, if she has to have an operation. It is important to let the doctor – especially the anaesthetist – know whether she has eaten or drunk anything before or after her accident. He will also want to know about any bad reactions to anaesthetics in your family.

Tests

Your child may have to have a variety of tests once she arrives in hospital, so that the doctors can start to put all the pieces of the jigsaw together, and find out exactly what is the matter. Or – if she has had an accident – to find out what blood group she is, so that if she needs it, she can have the correct blood given to her. (All blood transfusions now are AIDS tested and should be quite safe.) To do this, the doctor will take some blood from her vein using a needle and syringe. The child will feel a small scratch which might hurt a bit.

The doctor may want to take a specimen of her urine. If she is very small or very ill, the nurses will stick a plastic bag over the urethra (the hole where the urine comes out – see Chapter 2 on How the Body Works) and collect the urine once she has passed it into the bag. (With boys it is easier. They stick a plastic bag over the penis.)

If she has been badly injured or needs some emergency surgery, the doctor may put up a 'drip'. This is attached to a needle he gently slides into the child's vein and which is then left there – it is held in place by sticking plaster. This is then attached to a bottle of fluid (it might at some stage be blood) which is literally dripped into the vein.

If the doctor is going to put a 'drip' needle into the child's vein for any reason – NOT the most pleasant experience – he will almost certainly numb the skin first so that it doesn't hurt. One popular way of doing this is by using the 'magic' EMLA cream ('magic' because it stops it hurting!). Some hospitals use it all the time whenever a child has to have these sorts of injections, because they feel that the comfort of the child is the most important thing of all.

She may have to have an X-ray, if they think she has broken a bone. Women, including teenagers, who might be pregnant – even a few days late – must tell the X-ray technician. X-rays can kill or deform a foetus. You might want to be with your child at *any* examination which might upset her. But again, you may feel that – for whatever reason – you are not able to do this. Explain how you feel to the nurses and come in to see the child when you are able.

A doctor may come and listen to the child's chest with a stethoscope – particularly if she is going to have an operation. The anaesthetist will always do this before she goes to the operating theatre, because this doctor needs to make sure that the child is fit enough to have surgery.

If your child is going to stay in hospital, she will almost certainly be given the 'once-over' by the paediatrician to make sure there are no other illnesses which might make things worse. This will mean listening to her chest – even though the anaesthetist might be doing this as well – looking at her ears, nose and throat, checking her blood pressure and taking her pulse and temperature.

This doctor will also take a 'history'. In other words, he will ask the child – if she is able, or old enough to tell him – what happened and what she is feeling like. It would be helpful if you were there too, as he will almost certainly want to ask you some questions as well. However, if he is asking your child the questions, try to let her answer if you can. He is asking *her* and *not* you, so that he can get a better understanding of what is going on from the child's point of view.

If your child has come in as an emergency, you won't have had time to prepare her. The ward may have some books about going into hospital written in children's language that she can easily understand, and which you and she can read together. It might help her to voice the questions which may be swimming around in her head but which she may be too frightened to ask. (If by any chance she is going to be in hospital for a long time, you may want to send for the Action for Sick Children book list – see page 24.)

If your child is going to have an operation

Ask the nurse planning your child's care if you can go with her to the anaesthetic room to stay with her until she is asleep. Most hospitals not only allow this, but positively encourage parents to be there at what may be a rather frightening and bewildering time. (Your child may have been admitted to a hospital that is not too keen to let parents do this. It is then up to you to try to persuade them to allow you to be with your child.)

This also applies when she is 'coming round' from the anaesthetic after the operation. It is obviously nicer for the child if you are the first person she sees when she opens her eyes – but, having said that, you might not be able to do this. You mustn't worry or feel guilty about it, if you can't. The nurses will do *nearly* as good a job!

After the operation your child will be re-admitted to the ward until she is fit enough to go home. If she goes to the ward she will either go as a 'day case', which means she will just stay until the end of the day, or as an in-patient, in which case she will be allowed to go home as quickly as it is *safely* possible. If for some reason you cannot stay with your child in hospital, you might like to talk to her special nurse about her likes and dislikes.

Doctors now want to get children home as soon as they can so that they can be looked after by their parents (with maybe out-patient or community support), and not stay in a strange place, with strange people looking after them and strange bugs that they can easily pick up which make them worse than they were before they were admitted to hospital. There may be other reasons why the hospital wants to send them home, so make sure you feel your child is well enough and *you* feel confident to look after her. You must feel able to take the child back to hospital if you are worried, so ask for their direct line telephone number. You will also need enough pain-killers to make her comfortable until she's seen again by the doctors.

You might not feel able to look after your child at home, so talk to the doctor or the nurses about why you feel you can't manage and they will try and help you. It may also be difficult to stay or visit your child in hospital – if you are a single parent for instance. Again, try if you can to talk to the doctor or nurse in charge of your child, or ask if you can see someone you can talk to in confidence. They will understand how worried and guilty you may be feeling and will do all they can to help. Whatever else you do, don't try to keep these problems to yourself – you need to share the burden when you have a sick or injured child in hospital.

If you know someone who is not British or whose English is not very good, and their child has been taken to hospital in an emergency, they will probably feel even more anxious than those of us who understand roughly what is going on. They may want someone to interpret for them. If you can't do this they may want to take someone with them who can help. *Don't be afraid to ask for this for them.* As you know there are now lots of people in the same position and hospitals are usually geared up to deal with it; and if they are not, they should be! Some hospitals have leaflets printed in different languages which explain what goes on in that hospital and what you are expected to do.

If you are a parent with a disability and your child is brought to hospital, your anxieties may be quite different – apart from worrying about whether your child is going to be all right. In an emergency, you are not going to start quibbling about which hospital they are going to take your child to – you just want to get her to a place where they can deal quickly and efficiently with her accident or illness. However, if your child has to stay in hospital and they don't have the facilities you need to be able to visit her – such as a lift to take you up to the ward – or the journey is too difficult for you, the medical staff might be able to transfer her to a more suitable hospital, if there is a bed available.

For further information about the problems of having a child in hospital, contact:

Action for Sick Children
Argyle House, 29-31 Euston Road, London NW1 2SD.
Tel. 071 833 2041
This organisation used to be known as NAWCH, National Association for the Welfare of Children in Hospital. They are trying to get together a fully-staffed Parent Advice Service, but at the moment will supply excellent *written* information to help you if your child is going into hospital. They also have a very good children's book list.

HOW THE BODY WORKS

2

BREATHING SYSTEM

Air is breathed in through the **nose** and **mouth**. When air is breathed in through the nose, the tiny hairs and sticky mucus in the nostrils act as a filter and trap much of the dirt and dust that is in the air, before it travels further into the air passages. The next line of defence is the **tonsils**, two almond-shaped glands sitting on either side of the mouth where it meets the throat. The tonsils act as 'bouncers' by fighting infection entering the throat and stop it from spreading to other parts of the breathing system.

Most children breathe through their noses although some breathe through their mouths, particularly at night. If the nose is blocked (because of a cold, for instance) you may need to give him something to ease his breathing (see pages 203-204 on Coughs and Colds) and to stop mouth breathing from becoming a habit. (If your child breathes through his mouth a lot, or if he snores at night, take him to your GP just to check that his **adenoids** – the two fleshy glands sitting at the back of the throat – are not blocking his airway in any way.)

When air is breathed in it passes over the **epiglottis**. This is a small flap of cartilage which stands upright behind the tongue at the entrance to the **larynx**. The epiglottis immediately closes off the air passages when you eat or drink, so that you don't choke when you swallow. The air then passes through the larynx which is found at the front of the neck where it sticks out – more in boys than girls, particularly after puberty. The larynx is also called the Adam's apple or the voice box and this is exactly what it is – a sort of box made up of cartilage and muscle. It is just one of the many areas around a child's ear, nose and throat that may become inflamed and swollen when he is little. You can tell if this has happened because the child's breathing may become difficult and noisy (see Chapter 10 on Croup).

As air passes through the larynx, sounds are made by the air passing over the vocal cords as they vibrate. These sounds are how we communicate with one another – it's our voice! As the child grows, so does the larynx and as it does, the voice gets deeper.

The air then passes on into the windpipe or **trachea**. This is the ridged pipe that you can feel going down the front of the neck. The trachea branches into two tubes called the left and right main **bronchi**

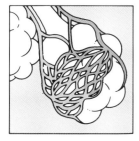

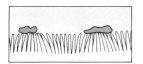

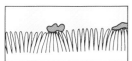

which lead to the **lungs**.

Each lung is a spongy mass of blood vessels and air passages. The smallest air tubes are called **bronchioles** at the ends of which are tiny sacs called **alveoli** which look like hollow bunches of tiny grapes. This is where carbon dioxide (waste gas) is swapped for oxygen, as the blood is pumped back into the lungs from other parts of the body. The oxygen-rich blood then circulates around the body and the carbon dioxide (waste gas) is breathed out.

It is this exchange of gases that is so important to keep going artificially if the child stops breathing for any reason. Parents should 'breathe for the child' so that oxygen can get to his brain as quickly as possible (see Chapter 3 on ABC Resuscitation Routine).

Tiny hairs called **cilia** line these airways and move dirt up and out preventing most of it from entering the lungs and causing infection.

The whole breathing system depends on a large dome-shaped muscle called the **diaphragm**, which forms the bottom of the chest cavity. It is the moving of the diaphragm up and down that forces the lungs to fill up with air and empty again, as we breathe.

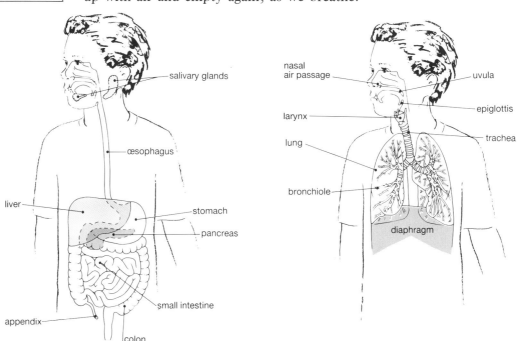

THE DIGESTIVE (EATING AND WASTE) SYSTEM

The digestive system breaks down food into tiny particles which seep into the blood stream through the digestive system and are used by the body. The breaking-down process starts very quickly once something has been eaten or drunk, and just as the good things are taken out of the food and sent around the body in the blood, so can the bad.

The **mouth** is a small factory. Once food or drink (or any other substance) goes into the mouth it starts to prepare the food for the stomach. The **teeth** chew the food up and as they do so saliva (spit) is mixed with it. **Saliva** contains chemicals, called **enzymes**, which start to break down the food. The chewed food is swallowed down the food pipe, called the **oesophagus**, and passes into the **stomach**. Whenever you eat or drink, the **epiglottis** – a small flap of cartilage which stands upright behind the tongue at the entrance to the throat – immediately closes off the air passages, so that you don't choke when you swallow.

Some substances, however, particularly drugs, start to get into the child's blood stream *from the mouth* – in other words, before they even reach the stomach. (Some drugs are made specially in this way.)

When the food enters the stomach, strong muscles squeeze and churn it and it is broken down further and digested by gastric juices containing enzymes in the stomach. Meanwhile the entrance to the stomach is held tightly shut, to stop the food from moving back up the oesophagus. (Of course, when a child is sick, this process is reversed and the food is forced out of the stomach and through the mouth.) The broken-down food then moves into the **small intestine** and is moved forwards through the digestive system by a series of strong muscular pushing and thrusting movements called **peristalsis** (rather like squeezing a tube of toothpaste downwards).

Most of the nourishment 'soaks' into the blood stream from the small intestine. This blood then goes to the parts of the body that need it most. (Remember, the digestive system can't tell if the child has swallowed food or poison. The **liver**, which acts as a food processing plant, may not be able to cope with a poisonous substance and it will pass into the child's blood stream.)

The liver also stores some of the nourishment, in the form of glucose (sugar), taken from the tiny particles of food in the blood. The **pancreas** usually checks the amount of glucose that gets into the blood stream. It makes hormones which trigger the liver to release more or less glucose, depending on what the child needs. One of these hormones is insulin. In diabetes, the pancreas is not able to produce the right amount of insulin for the body and the child has to be given insulin artificially, almost always by injection. (See Chapter 11 on Diabetes.)

From the small intestine the 'food' (although it doesn't look much like it now) enters the **large intestine** (the gut) where the last of the goodies, the minerals and water are taken out and pass into the blood stream.

The waste products are anything the body doesn't want, and these make their way into the **rectum**, the last part of the large intestine. When the child feels ready to do so, he pushes the stool out through the anus (the back-passage), when he goes to the toilet.

Diarrhoea is caused by food passing through the gut too quickly, not leaving enough time for it to be digested and the liquid to soak into the blood (see page 26). Constipation on the other hand is caused by food remaining in the gut for longer than it should, and too much water from the stool soaking into the body. The stool becomes harder and it is more difficult for the child to pass when he goes to the toilet.

BLOOD AND CIRCULATION

It is important to understand the difference between adults' and children's circulation. Children have less blood in their bodies. The average adult carries about 8 pints (5 litres) whereas an average five-year-old carries only *half* that amount. A one-year-old baby carries about 2 pints (800ml). So any accident where the child bleeds a lot is going to be dangerous.

Blood travels through a one-way circulatory transport system of **arteries** and **veins** and supplies the body with food and oxygen. Blood is filled with **oxygen** in the **lungs** and the oxygen-rich blood is then pumped by the **heart** through the arteries around the body. (If a child has an accident it is very important that he is put in a position, usually lying down, to help the blood get to the vital centres of his body – the brain, lungs, heart and kidneys. See Chapter 6 on Bleeding.)

If the child has an accident and the heart stops his circulation must be kept going until he gets expert medical help to restart his heart. Circulation can be continued artificially by pressing on the child's chest, which squeezes the heart from the outside of the body. *This technique of resuscitation is vital for parents to know in order to save a child's life.* (See Chapter 3 on ABC Resuscitation Routine.)

The arteries get smaller as they move away from the heart. They branch into tiny pathways called **capillaries** which feed and nourish every part of the child's body. It is through these that carbon dioxide is swapped for oxygen. The veins then bring the blood back again to the heart and lungs – the body having used some of the oxygen – and the process starts all over again.

Blood is a red, thick, sticky fluid that is made up of liquid and solid parts. There are three solid parts which float around in the fluid – **red cells, white cells** and **platelets**. The red cells – there are about 200 million of them in one drop of blood – contain **haemoglobin** (a red chemical which carries oxygen), so the redder the blood, the more oxygen it is carrying. Red blood is called **arterial** blood, coming straight from the lungs and carried to the body by the arteries. When the oxygen has been used up on its journey around the body the blood starts to go blue. This **venous** blood is then pumped back to the lungs through the veins for a 'top up' of oxygen.

White cells carry chemicals which fight infection coming into the child's body. Platelets contain a chemical (fibrin) which helps the blood to clot when it flows out of the blood vessels onto the surface of the skin.

Plasma is the straw-coloured liquid part of blood. It carries nourishment to, and waste from, the body and it also carries anti-bodies which fight infection.

There is a constant cleansing and stocking up of the child's blood. Waste products are carried away in the blood, and are got rid of through the body's waste systems. The **lungs** take out waste gases – carbon dioxide and some water vapour – which are breathed out through the nose and mouth. The **kidneys** take out waste fluid – urine – which is passed out of the body through the bladder and the urethra.

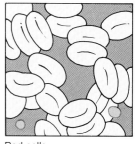

Red cells.

Bleeding is always serious because it cuts down the amount of blood going round the child's body, causing his blood pressure to fall and the child to go into shock. If a child has an accident and he bleeds *into* the body rather than outside it (that is, he has internal bleeding), there is a danger that the blood could ooze into a cavity such as the chest or the skull. It can then do a lot of damage by pressing on the lung, the brain or whatever vital organ is in that particular space (see Chapter 6 on Bleeding).

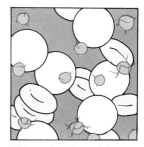

White cells help to fight infection with platelets.

There are four main blood groups (rather like fingerprints, every person's is slightly different): A, B, AB and O. Blood is also described as being Rhesus positive or Rhesus negative (this classification is named after the Rhesus monkey on which scientists did special laboratory tests to find anti-bodies). Your child's blood group may be written like this: O Rhesus +ve.

If a child bleeds from a wound or has to have an operation, he may have to have a **blood transfusion**.

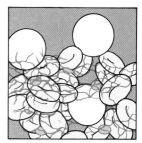

Red cells bind together with the help of fibrin from platelets to form clot.

Once in hospital, the doctor will take a sample of his blood to have it cross-matched for group and Rhesus-factor. This means the laboratory staff test your child's blood against the blood that might have to be given to him. This is to make sure that his body will accept the 'new' blood he is given.

ALL blood is tested (at the time it is given by the donor) to make sure it does not contain the AIDS virus.

URINARY SYSTEM

This is a filtering system for the body. The blood has to be constantly cleaned, otherwise it would get clogged up with all the dangerous waste products that the body doesn't want. The fluid waste is made into **urine** in the **kidneys**. There are two kidneys, right and left, situated high up at the back of the abdomen. From there the urine runs through two tubes, called the **ureters**, into a pouch called the **bladder**. When this gets full, the child gets a message from the brain that the bladder needs to be emptied by passing urine.

When urine is passed into the toilet it comes out of a tube called the **urethra**. This tube is slightly different in boys and girls. In boys, the urethra comes down the length of the penis and is the same tube that is

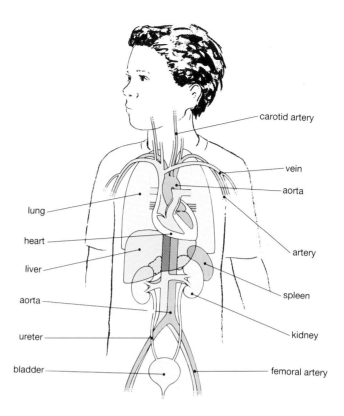

used when they pass sperm (ejaculate). In girls, the urethra is much shorter and is inside the body. It runs *separately*, on the top of the vagina. The entrance to it is found just in front of the vaginal opening.

MUSCLES AND BONES

Muscles

There are about 600 **muscles** in a child's body – all at different stages of development – which help children to move about. Most muscles work in pairs and each pair is attached to two bones at either end, between which is a **joint**. The muscles are joined to the bones by **tendons**. These are strong, sometimes quite long, cords which take the slack when the muscle is moved. With the help of the tendons, muscles can move the bone up or down, depending on what **nerve** signals are being sent from the brain. Some work all the time, such as the heart – these are made in a special way to prevent them from getting tired – others work only when the child wants them to.

Most muscles get tired (this particularly applies to children). When a child moves a muscle (which he does all the time when simply walking about, and more so in exercise) he uses up a lot of energy and, after a while, gets tired. When he exercises, his muscles will grow stronger and he will become fitter and tire less easily.

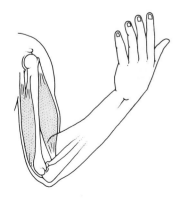

Bones

A child has 206 **bones** in his body – half of these are in his hands and feet! Bones keep the body shape and also protect what is inside. So the skull protects the brain, the ribcage the heart and lungs and so on.

It is important to know what a child's bones look like so that you can understand how best to look after them when they get damaged. Each bone is made up of three parts, a hard outer layer made mainly of calcium salts (that's why foods rich in calcium, such as cheese, yogurt and liver, are so good for growing children), a spongy but hard layer and a soft jelly-like centre which contains the bone marrow and is full of tiny blood vessels and nerves.

However hard each individual bone seems, the whole skeleton is remarkably flexible and is capable of a huge range of movements.

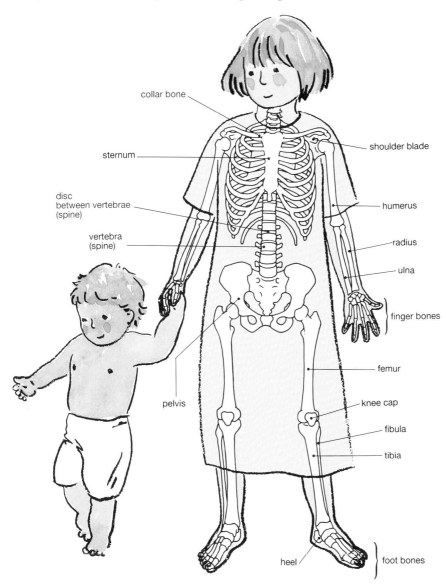

collar bone

shoulder blade

sternum

disc
between vertebrae
(spine)

humerus

vertebra
(spine)

radius

ulna

finger bones

femur

pelvis

knee cap

fibula

tibia

heel

foot bones

31

Near each end of every bone are bands of **cartilage** and it is from here that the bone grows. When a child breaks a bone, a **callus** binds the bone together making it whole again. *It is always very important for a child with a fracture to get the medical attention he needs quickly.* The only way to find out for sure if he has broken something, is to take the child to hospital to have an **X-ray** picture of the bone.

If the fracture is left undiscovered and not treated immediately (see Chapter 18 on Fractures and Bone Injuries) then the callus starts forming anyway – it doesn't realise that the pieces of broken bone may be overlapping, misshapen or not quite in their right place. If it is left untreated the bone may be shorter, or look an odd shape, once it is healed.

In a young child with a bad fracture, there is a chance that the growth area in the healing bone may be damaged and the bone may not grow as well as the others.

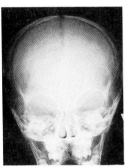

HEAD

In a new-born baby the head makes up about one quarter of the total body length. The outside bony skull is made up of the **base** and the **vault** (the bottom and the top). It is a box into which the brain and the fluid which surrounds and protects it are packed.

Babies are born with two 'soft spots' (the **fontanelles**) at the top of their heads, where the bones of the skull are not quite joined. (This helps the baby ease through the birth canal, as the soft spot helps the bones of the skull to overlap slightly, making the head smaller than it would otherwise be. Sometimes, particularly if the birth has taken a long time, the bones take a few days to get back to normal. This is called moulding.) The fontanelles have usually closed up by the time the child is eighteen months old.

The brain

The **brain** lies within the skull surrounded and protected by a crystal-clear fluid, called CSF (Cerebro-Spinal Fluid). The brain is the main part of the central nervous system and is responsible for and co-ordinates all our movements and thoughts, including memory, emotions and language. The brain stem at the base of the brain, leading to the spinal cord, is responsible for automatic processes such as breathing and digestion. Each side of the brain has different functions. If the brain gets damaged, in an accident for instance, the child may be unable to do the things that the injured side of the brain is responsible for. The brain uses the nerves as its messenger network to communicate what it wants to do to the rest of the body (see Nerves below).

The head contains the body's main sense organs – the eyes and ears, the taste buds of the tongue and the nose for smell. These sense organs

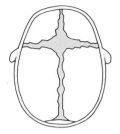

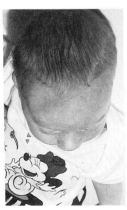

Moulding of the fontanelles. This is what a child's head will look like after a long labour. The soft bones overlap to ease the baby's passage through the birth canal.

pick up information and send it back to the brain by tiny electrical signals. The brain can then send messages to the nerves and muscles, through the **spinal cord** (found in the backbone, or spine, running down the back) telling the body what action to take.

The mouth

The **mouth** takes in food – and anything else that the child wishes to put into it! It also contains the **tongue** and **teeth** which, with the help of saliva (spit) from the salivary glands, enable the child to chew and start to digest food. The teeth and tongue also help the child make the first sounds of speech.

Babies are usually born without teeth. Within three or four years, toddlers develop twenty milk teeth. Once the child reaches about six years old, these teeth start to fall out and the adult teeth eventually develop and replace the milk teeth. By the time he is about fourteen years old he will have about thirty-two of these. If you look at an X-ray of a ten-year-old child's mouth, you will see the milk teeth with the adult teeth underneath them waiting to come through.

The **tongue** is a muscle. It cannot be swallowed, but when a child is unconscious, it can flop back and mould itself to the back of the throat, which can obstruct breathing (see page 39).

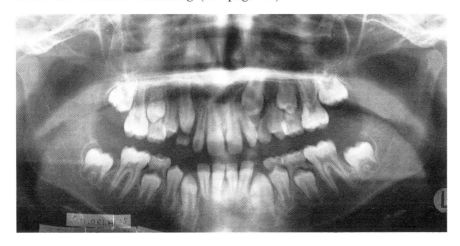

X-ray of a nine-year-old's mouth. See the adult teeth underneath the milk teeth.

The nose

The **nose** is divided into two nostrils by a sheet of cartilage and thin bone called the **nasal septum**. Each nostril filters, warms and wets the air before it travels down the air passages. On either side of the nose are two **sinuses** – or hollow spaces – which sometimes fill up with and become blocked by infected mucus.

The nose is continuous with the back of the mouth, so anything going into the mouth or nose reaches the same place at the back of the throat. This includes air and food (or anything else the child puts into his mouth or nose).

At the back of the throat are the two **Eustachian tubes** which join

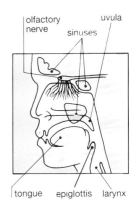

olfactory nerve | uvula | sinuses
tongue epiglottis larynx

the throat to the middle ear chamber. It is because the nose is actually *joined* to the ear by this tube that children can get ear infections after getting a runny nose or cold.

The ear

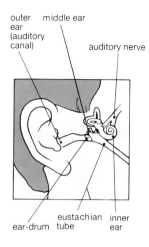

outer ear (auditory canal)   middle ear

auditory nerve

ear-drum   eustachian tube   inner ear

The **ear** collects sound waves from the air. They are processed through the three parts of the ear, the outer, middle and inner ear. The outer ear is the bit you can see, in the centre of which is a small hole leading into the delicate inside parts that collect sound waves and send them to the brain. The middle ear starts at the ear-drum – any sound that goes into the ear makes this drum vibrate. These vibrations go through three tiny bones to the inner ear where hairs line a fluid-filled tube called the **cochlea**. These move to the vibrations of the sound and trigger electrical nerve signals to the brain which tells the child what the sound is. If the sounds are too close *and* too loud (like personal stereos), the child can become deaf.

The inner ear is also responsible for balance. Too much noise or unusual fast movement can upset its delicate balance mechanism. That is why when children twiz round and round for a few seconds or more, on a 'Big Dipper' for instance, they become dizzy and are sometimes sick.

The eye

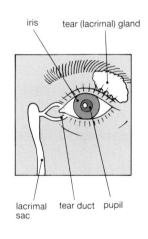

iris   tear (lacrimal) gland

lacrimal sac   tear duct   pupil

The **eye** is a delicate, complicated and amazing piece of engineering. Each eye is protected by a bony socket. The eyelids protect the eye from the outside and moisten them every time the child blinks. The eye is moved around by six muscles which keep the eyeball facing the way it should. The back of the eye is connected to the brain by the **optic nerve**.

The **conjunctiva** is the transparent outside covering of the eye which is extremely sensitive and can sometimes become infected. At the inner corner of each eye are the **tear ducts** which are small tubes leading from the eye to the back of the nose. The **pupil** is the black circle in the middle of the muscular, coloured (blue, brown or green) **iris**. The edges of the pupil look as if they are elasticated, and in a way they are. The pupil is relaxed and wide open in dim light or in the dark, but in bright light the iris muscle tenses up and the pupil becomes smaller. If a child is deeply unconscious, or if he has some brain infection or damage, the pupils may not react to light, that is they will stay the same size whether it is dark or light. This is a serious warning sign.

The **cornea** is the front window through which the light passes into the eyeball. The **lens** lies behind the pupil and focuses light on the **retina**, at the back of the eye. The retina works like a video camera but it takes the picture upside down and sends the message through the optic nerve to the brain.

SKIN

Skin is waterproof and protects the child's body against poisons and injury. Infection and disease usually only get in when the skin is broken. Skin helps to control body temperature, but babies and younger children can't sweat or shiver and need help to keep warm or cool, by putting them in appropriate clothing to control their temperature (see Chapter 21 on Hypothermia and Hyperthermia).

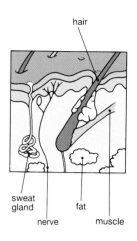

sweat gland

nerve

hair

fat

muscle

Skin contains an elastic material which makes it stretchy. It is made up of cells and has lots of layers, the top layer is constantly being replaced from underneath – most house dust is actually dead skin cells which are rubbed off whenever the child moves about. Skin contains **melanin**, a dark pigment, which protects the skin from the harmful rays of the sun. The darker the skin, the better chance the child has of being protected from sun damage.

Except for the palms of the hands and the soles of the feet, skin is covered with hair – some so fine that you can hardly see it – which also helps to control the child's temperature by trapping air.

The underneath layers of skin contain sweat and oil glands. In later childhood and adolescence these may become active and the child may need advice about diet, washing and treating spots.

NERVES

Nerves sense how the body is functioning. They send messages to and from the brain telling the child when and how to move, when he is feeling pain or pleasure, or if he is hungry or tired. Messages are also sent through the nerves from the bones, muscles, skin and other organs telling the child if something is wrong, e.g. when he has hurt himself. Nerves take messages to or from the central nervous system and are co-ordinated by the spinal cord and brain. They have a million different functions but we rarely notice them until they go wrong. If nerves get injured they are poor growers and repairers. In other words, if a child has an accident the last things to mend are often the nerves. If they are seriously damaged they may not be repaired and this may result in a permanent numbness or weakness.

3 ABC RESUSCITATION ROUTINE

The most important first aid for you to know is how to bring a child who has stopped breathing back to life. This whole process is called 'resuscitation' and it is important to do it in a special order which is recognised all over the world.

This international checklist is in four parts. You must know each part to get the child out of danger and maybe even save her life:

1 Is there any further **DANGER** to you or your child? If not:

2 Check **A** for **AIRWAY** (is it clear?)

3 Check **B** for **BREATHING** (is she breathing?)

4 Check **C** for **CIRCULATION** (is her heart beating?)

If your child is having trouble breathing or stops breathing YOU MUST START YOUR ABC RESUSCITATION ROUTINE IMMEDIATELY *even* if she is seriously injured or very ill. It may mean, for instance, moving her with badly broken limbs or even a spinal injury (where you would normally *never* move her). Resuscitation is MORE IMPORTANT than anything else.

WITHOUT THIS RESUSCITATION ROUTINE SHE WILL DIE.

DANGER

There is one sensible and often life-saving precaution to take before you can even think of ABC and that is to look for danger – danger to you and added danger to the child you are trying to help.

Let us imagine that you come into the room to find your child lying unconscious on the floor. You quickly look round to see what has happened and you find, for example, that she is touching a rather blackened plug. The chances are that she has given herself an electric shock and if you touch her, you will get a shock too.

So, no matter how you may feel, you must remove her from the supply BEFORE touching her. You can do this by knocking the wire or plug away from her with something that does not conduct electricity, such as a broom-handle or a rolled-up newspaper; or by turning off the electricity supply at the mains. (Do you know where your mains elec-

EMERGENCY BODY POINTS

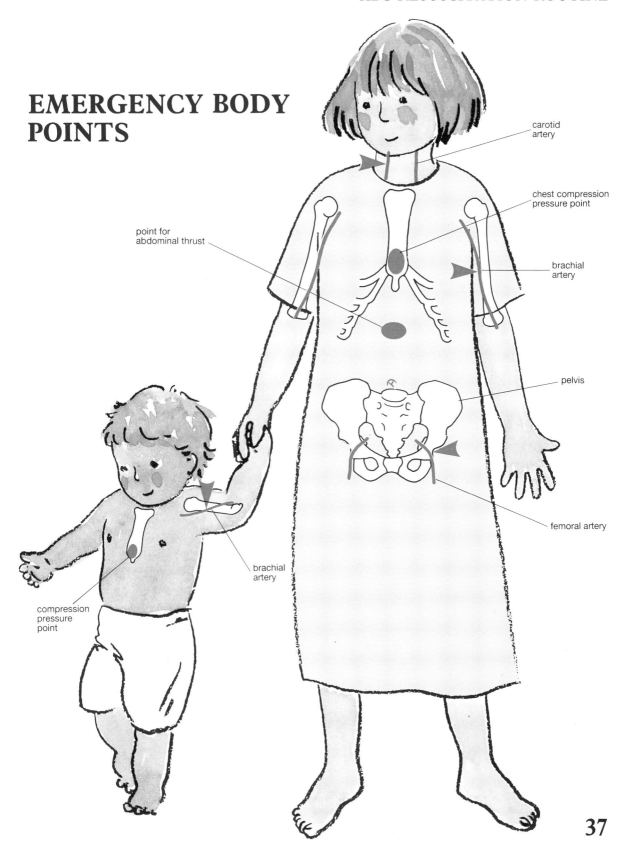

carotid
artery

chest compression
pressure point

point for
abdominal thrust

brachial
artery

pelvis

brachial
artery

femoral artery

compression
pressure
point

tricity switch is and, more to the point, how to turn it off? There may be more than one switch.) As soon as you have done this, you can begin your Resuscitation Routine – but not before (see Chapter 15 on Electric Shock).

There will be different dangers in every situation. You have to assess them quickly and make sure that you know how to avoid them. For instance, if your child is in a road accident try to get someone to direct the traffic away from her. You can then give her the emergency treatment she needs to keep her safe until the ambulance arrives.

If she is in danger from an unsafe building, for instance, you may have to move the child *before* you treat her, even though this is not ideal. If your child is drowning and you feel you cannot reach her safely, SHOUT FOR HELP before you start to rescue her.

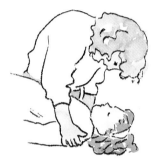

So always look out for DANGER before you begin any resuscitation. Once you know the surroundings are safe, you can look after the child more effectively.

First you need to know if she is CONSCIOUS. One way to find out is to shake the child gently and shout, 'Are you OK – what has happened?' If she doesn't respond, YOU NEED TO GET MEDICAL HELP URGENTLY. Don't try to cope all by yourself. If you can, get someone to call for an ambulance by dialling 999. Tell them the child is unconscious.

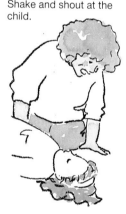

Shake and shout at the child.

However, if she is still a baby you can't ask, 'Are you OK?' but just shake her and shout at her. If she is conscious she will respond to you.

While the ambulance is on its way to you the emergency operator will take you through the things that you must do to save your child's life. Try to listen carefully to what he or she is telling you.

If you don't have a phone, go to the front doorstep and shout for help. Get someone to phone urgently for an ambulance – make sure that whoever is phoning tells them the number of your house or flat and how to find it easily.

WHAT TO DO

Start your ABC.

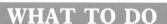

A for **AIRWAY** (is it clear?)

B for **BREATHING** (is she breathing?)

C for **CIRCULATION** (is her heart beating?)

A FOR AIRWAY

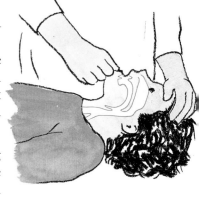

1   Carry the child to a table or some other firm surface. It might have to be the floor, but you won't have as much control there as you would at table level. With one hand on the forehead, and the first finger of the other hand on the bony part of the chin, tilt the head back, grip the chin and lift it forward.

2   Look inside the mouth to see if there is anything obvious blocking the airway. If it's the tongue, for instance, when you pull up the chin to free the airway there may be a choking sound and you will know immediately that she has started breathing again. The child can't swallow her tongue but when she is unconscious it can block the airway (see Chapter 2 on How the Body Works). In a baby the neck is much shorter and chubbier than in older children. You need to be careful not to push the head too far back. On the other hand, it is vital that the short airway is fully extended. Put your hand under the shoulders for better support.

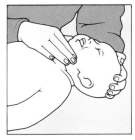

3   If there is a lump of vomit, food or small object that you can see, then scoop it out if you can by doing a quick 'finger-sweep'. If, however, you can't get it out immediately, don't poke. (DON'T stick your finger blindly down her throat, you could do more damage by pushing whatever it is further down.)

4   Turn the child over your knee and slap five times between the shoulder blades. Check that nothing has come flying out of the mouth (see Chapter 8 on Choking).

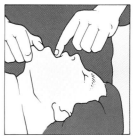

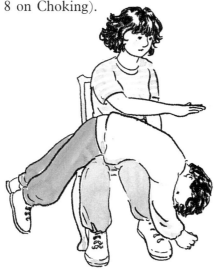

5   Check the nostrils. Small children and babies tend to breathe through their nostrils, and if they are blocked this can make a difficult situation a lot worse. If, however, you feel there is nothing obvious blocking her airway, move quickly to B.

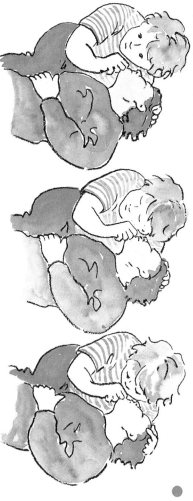

B FOR BREATHING

If breathing stops there is no oxygen getting to the brain. *Within three minutes* the brain cells begin to die. It is vital that you take urgent action to restart the child's breathing as soon as you possibly can.

The three things to remember are:

1 **LOOK**
2 **LISTEN** } for breathing
3 **FEEL**

Do all of these by placing your ear over the child's mouth to:

1 **LOOK** along the outline of her chest, to see if her chest is rising and falling, as it normally does when she breathes.

2 **LISTEN** for breathing sounds.

3 **FEEL** for breath coming out of her mouth or nostrils onto the side of your face. Spend about five seconds doing this. Her breath may be very shallow and you may not be able to feel it at first. If breathing has stopped, then you must act quickly and breathe *for* the child in order to fill the air sacs of the lungs with air (see Chapter 2 on How the Body Works). This is called Artificial Respiration. If you are not sure whether or not her breathing has stopped, start to breathe for her anyway.

When you are breathing for a child REMEMBER to:

● Be gentle yet firm enough to tilt the head back, lifting the chin upwards so that the airway opens – otherwise no air can get through.

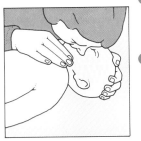

● Cover the child's mouth, or mouth and nose if the child is under four years old, with your mouth and breathe into her deeply enough to fill the air sacs at the bottom of the lungs.

● If you do not cover the nose with your mouth as you breathe into her mouth, then squeeze the nostrils with your finger and thumb at the same time to stop the air escaping. It doesn't matter which method you use, do whatever feels comfortable depending on the age and size of the child, as long as you stop the air escaping as you are breathing it in.

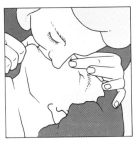

● GIVE FIVE SEPARATE BREATHS, each enough to make her chest rise as if she is taking a deep breath. Take your mouth away after each breath. As you breathe into her, LOOK along the outside of her chest, to see if it is rising each time. If it is, this means that the air you breathe in is travelling down the airway and into the tiny air sacs in the lungs. It is only by reaching these air sacs that the exchange of gases (oxygen and carbon dioxide) can take place.

There is a difference between resuscitating babies and resuscitating children.

When you are breathing for a baby, remember three things:

1 It is better to cover the *mouth and nose* to get a better flow of air into the airway.

2 Remember the neck is shorter, chubbier and more fragile. Be gentle, yet firm enough to tilt the head back so the airway is open, otherwise no air can get through.

3 Blow until you see the chest start to rise.

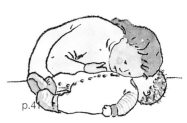
Blow until you see the chest rise.

Remember: DON'T BLOW TOO HARD. There is a danger that air could be blown into her tummy, causing the food inside to spill over into the lungs.

If the chest does not rise the most likely reason is that the airway is not fully open, so *look again* at the position of the head and see if you can gently lift the chin up or tilt the head back a bit more. It is only by adjusting the airway and straightening out any kinks that you can get the correct position and allow air to pass through more easily. Alternatively, there may be something stuck in the airway so use the choking sequence (see Chapter 8 on Choking).

C FOR CIRCULATION

After giving the first five breaths into the child's mouth (or, if the child is small, mouth *and nose*), you must immediately check to see if the heart is beating. There is no point in breathing for her *if the oxygen is not being circulated around the body*.

The whole purpose of resuscitation is to KEEP THE BRAIN ALIVE. Whether *you* do this or the *heart* does it, doesn't matter. What matters is getting the blood circulating again urgently and as efficiently as possible.

The way to find out is to feel for the pulse. The best place to find the pulse in a child over one year old is at the **carotid artery**. This passes either side of the windpipe in the neck and can be felt by pressing two forefingers gently at this point.

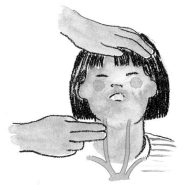
Feeling for the neck pulse (carotid).

The carotid pulse is the strongest in the body. When a child has an accident she is often shocked, and it is essential to have the strongest pulse at your fingertips. Check the pulse for five seconds.

It may be difficult to find the neck pulse in a baby, because the neck tends to be short and chubby. The easier one, therefore, is the **brachial pulse**. This is found on the inside of the upper arm, midway between the elbow and the shoulder. Press your two forefingers gently towards the bone, while you hold the outside of the arm with your thumb.

Feeling for the arm pulse in a baby (brachial).

(It is a good idea to 'practise' on your own child, so that you know where the pulse is and what it feels like. It is often difficult to find a pulse in an emergency unless you are used to feeling it. You may think this is tempting fate – I just think it is sensible to practise.)

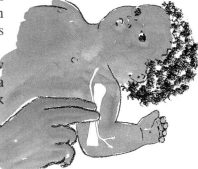

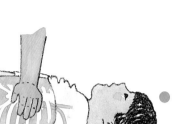

If she has *not* got a pulse and you have not called or phoned for help, this is the time to interrupt the Routine to do so.

If you cannot feel a pulse, you must begin chest compression (heart massage). This means pressing the child's chest so that the blood – with its vital oxygen – is pumped around the body and up to her brain. Hopefully the heart (about the size of her closed fist) will then start to beat again by itself.

For children over one year old

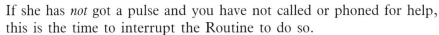

- Place the heel of one hand just below the nipple line in the middle of her chest and press down firmly, so that the pressure of your hand pushes the chest in about 1 to 1½ inches (2.5 to 3.5cm).

- Straighten your arm and hold your shoulders directly over the child's chest. This is terribly important because it puts you in the best position to press on the chest and get her heart started again.

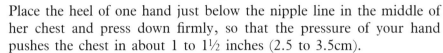

- PRESS FIRMLY FIVE TIMES at the rate of 100 beats per minute or three times every two seconds (that is, slightly quicker than one press every second).

- THEN GIVE THE CHILD ONE BREATH, using mouth-to-mouth (or in a small child, mouth-to-mouth-nose) breathing (see above, B for Breathing). Then repeat the whole Routine. Press her chest five times, then give her one breath.

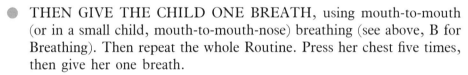

- If she is not breathing but has a pulse, continue to breathe for her giving a breath every three seconds. Keep checking her pulse. Continue until help arrives.

Babies

REMEMBER a baby's heart is about the same size as her tiny fist. Don't forget to ask yourself, how much pressure do I need to squash this heart down? Just press hard enough to get it started again – about ¾ of an inch (2cm).

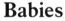

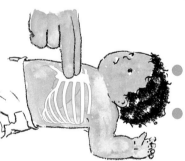

Use two forefingers at the point one finger-breadth below the nipple line.

Press five times, then give one breath.

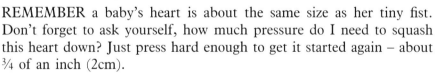

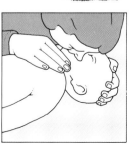

Remember, whether it is a baby or a child who stops breathing, the sooner you can begin resuscitation the better chance you have of saving her life.

You need to get expert medical help urgently. If you haven't done so already, call for an ambulance by dialling 999. Continue breathing for your child and giving her chest compressions. Tell the emergency operator what you are trying to do.

While the ambulance is on its way to you, they will take you through the Resuscitation Routine so that you don't feel that you are coping on your own with a child who isn't breathing.

KEEP RESUSCITATING UNTIL THE AMBULANCE ARRIVES.

Why babies stop breathing

There are a number of different reasons why your baby might stop breathing. Cot death, which kills one in 400 children between the ages of one month and one year, is the greatest single cause of infant death in the Western world. This is one reason why every parent or carer should know how to resuscitate a baby. You might get there too late, but if the baby has only just stopped breathing, you have a chance to save her life (see Chapter 9 on Cot Death).

If you think that your baby is ill, never hesitate to call the doctor. Doctors would rather see a baby the parent or carer thinks is ill, and isn't, than a very ill baby whose parents didn't realise and may have left it too late.

The *Safe and Sound* video of this technique may help you to understand it even better (see page 284 for details).

RECOVERY POSITION

If, at any stage of the ABC Resuscitation Routine, the child starts breathing again, roll her quickly but gently into the Recovery Position. Then, if she is sick, this position will stop her from inhaling her vomit and choking. It is important to put the child in this position in the following way:

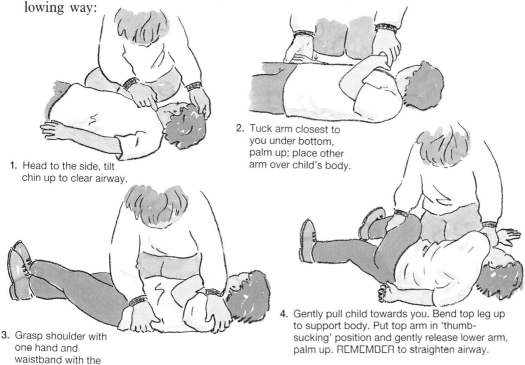

1. Head to the side, tilt chin up to clear airway.

2. Tuck arm closest to you under bottom, palm up; place other arm over child's body.

3. Grasp shoulder with one hand and waistband with the other.

4. Gently pull child towards you. Bend top leg up to support body. Put top arm in 'thumb-sucking' position and gently release lower arm, palm up. REMEMBER to straighten airway.

IN A SEVERE ACCIDENT OR ILLNESS, IT IS MORE LIKELY THAT A CHILD'S BREATHING WOULD STOP RATHER THAN HER HEART.

THE MOST IMPORTANT THING FOR ANYONE LOOKING AFTER A CHILD IN THIS SITUATION IS TO GET MEDICAL HELP AS QUICKLY AS YOU CAN.

THINK

- Have you managed to get some help? Try shouting out of the window or front door.
- Have you called the ambulance? Try to get someone to do this for you.
- Have you checked for DANGER?
- Shake and shout to the child to see if she is conscious.

IF THE CHILD BECOMES UNCONSCIOUS: be ready to start your ABC RESUSCITATION ROUTINE.

Now check   'A' for AIRWAY – is it clear?

IF SHE DOESN'T RESPOND: OPEN THE AIRWAY. Tilt the child's head back and lift her chin forward. REMEMBER babies' necks are chubbier and more fragile. **Be gentle yet firm enough to tilt head back so airway is open.**

Now check   'B' for BREATHING

LOOK
LISTEN } for breathing
FEEL

IF THE CHILD IS NOT BREATHING: BREATHE FOR THE CHILD. Cover her mouth, or nose and mouth, with your mouth. Give her FIVE separate breaths. Watch her chest rise with each breath. REMEMBER you need *less* breath for babies.

Now check   'C' for CIRCULATION

Is her heart beating? Check for the pulse. Feel the neck (or arm in a baby) for a pulse. **If there is no pulse and you haven't got help GET IT NOW.**

IF YOU CANNOT FEEL A PULSE: DO CHEST COMPRESSION. Feel for the right place – one finger-breadth below the nipple line. Press on the chest, at a rate of **100 presses per minute.**

For children over one year old: Use the 'heel' of one hand only, with your arm straight. **Press fifteen times to every two breaths** (so your hand presses in about 2.5-3.5cm or 1-1½ inches each time).

For babies: Use two fingers only and **press five times to one breath** (so your fingers press in about 2cm which is about ¾ of an inch, each time).

KEEP DOING THIS UNTIL THE AMBULANCE ARRIVES.

ALLERGIES

4

An allergy is the body's unnatural response to a substance which is usually absolutely harmless to most children. If a child is allergic to a substance and it is inhaled, eaten, touched or injected into the skin, it causes the child's body to react in an unusual way.

Most of the time childhood allergies are little more than a nuisance, sometimes they can make the child feel ill, but occasionally they can be extremely dangerous and may even be life-threatening. It is important for parents and carers to be aware of the difference.

There are two factors which need to be thought about. One is that if *you* had an allergy in childhood, your child will probably find something to be allergic to as well. The other is that a child can go along happily with something such as an antibiotic that he has taken in the past, or a plant that he may have touched loads of times before, when all of a sudden he will have a big allergic reaction to it. Allergic reactions are peculiar things and if the child looks as if he's having one, he probably IS, even if he hasn't reacted like this before.

There are dozens of types of reactions that a child might have to dozens of different allergens (things to which he might be allergic). The ones described below are those that need first aid treatment.

If he has eaten or swallowed something to which his body has taken a violent dislike, he will probably be sick some time over the next few hours (see Chapter 23 on Poisoning). If he is *allergic* to it, his body's reaction to it may be more immediate.

If your child is on a medicine, such as penicillin, and he starts to have 'allergic' symptoms you must stop the medicine immediately even though you will have been told to continue with it until the end of the course. Phone and speak to your doctor telling him what you have done and listen to what he wants you to do.

(Always check with your doctor about possible allergic reactions to a drug he may want your child to take – particularly if your child has had allergic reactions to anything before or if he has eczema or asthma.)

WHAT TO LOOK FOR

● He may start with an itching sensation of the lips, or he may have a general itch all over.

● He may develop a slight rash all over his body, or he may get very severe weals and swelling on some or all parts of his body – this is called urticaria or nettle-rash and is the body's way of attracting attention to the fact that it doesn't like what has been put in or near it.

45

- His lips, mouth and tongue might swell up, as may his hands or eyes.

- He may wheeze (see Chapter 5 on Asthma).

- Occasionally the swelling becomes so bad that it affects his breathing passages and the child could stop breathing. *This is a medical emergency. He will be terrified and the more frightened he is, the more difficult he will find it to breathe.*

- If, however, the food or substance is *beginning to be digested* before the body starts to reject it, the reaction is slower and not as dramatic, but could be just as serious. The first thing the child might do, for instance, is to complain of a 'colicky' tummy ache, often along with feeling sick, being sick or having diarrhoea. This is like food poisoning, but then the other symptoms mentioned above may begin to appear.

- The child might develop shock if all the symptoms are severe (see Chapter 27 on Shock).

REMEMBER – SHOCK LOOKS LIKE THIS

- His face may be very pale and grey-looking

- His skin may feel cold and clammy

- His pulse may feel fast and weak

- He may be frightened and fidgety

- He may be very thirsty

- He may yawn and 'gasp' for air

- He may say everything feels fuzzy

- He may become unconscious

WHAT TO DO

- If the tongue and throat swell up and the child has difficulty in breathing, prop him up on pillows, particularly if he is wheezy, or put him in a position that is most comfortable for him. The more comfortable you can make him the calmer he will be.

    If he becomes unconscious, quickly lie him down on a flat surface, and open his airway. Watch his breathing carefully. If it stops, start your ABC Resuscitation Routine immediately.

> **A** for **AIRWAY** (is it clear?)
>
> **B** for **BREATHING** (is he breathing?)
>
> **C** for **CIRCULATION** (is his heart beating?)

● Tell him what is happening and what you are trying to do. If you are dealing with a small child try not to show your panic.

● See if you can find someone to phone for an ambulance (see Chapter 1 on Preparation and Practical Issues). If you are on your own and you haven't got a telephone, get a neighbour to help you. But remember, do not leave the child alone.

● If you think he might be sick, roll him over into the Recovery Position.

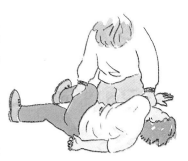

Prevention

There are some doctors who think that eating junk food might be one of the causes of an allergic reaction in some children, even though allergies to food only affect a very small number. If your child IS allergic to any particular food he – and you – will know about it quite quickly because the effect is usually dramatic. There are some foods which violently affect some children. These include shell-fish, eggs, dairy products, wheat, nuts, chocolate, and some berries such as strawberries.

If it is not immediately obvious, you need to know what makes your child react in an allergic way. He may need to see an allergy specialist who will try to find out which food is causing the problem. This doctor will need you to keep a list of all the things your child eats during the day, so that he and you will have more of an idea about what it is, when, or if, your child has a reaction.

He may then do some simple skin tests on your child, in hospital. It is very useful, and sometimes vital, for you to know if there is one particular thing from which he should keep away. If your child is sensitive to penicillin, for instance, he should wear a bracelet so that people will know that he must NOT have this drug, even in an emergency.

Alternatively you might like to try acupuncture, ideally combined with homoeopathy. The practitioners who use these alternative methods of healing, as long as they have been well recommended, often have great skills. Acupuncture can be very effective in treating some children with allergic disorders and *preventing them occurring again*, but it is slower to work than orthodox medicine. The results can be as good as the drugs your doctor may prescribe; sometimes they are much better.

For further information about allergies contact:

The British Allergy Foundation
St Bartholemew's Hospital, West Smithfield, London EC1A 7BE.

Alternatively you could contact the following organisations which only recommend registered acupuncturists and homoeopaths and ask them if any of the practitioners specialise in treating children:

The Council for Acupuncture
179 Gloucester Place, London NW1 6DX.
Tel. 071 724 5756

The Society of Homoeopaths
2 Artizan Road, Northampton NN1 4HU.
Tel. 0604 21400

You may like to read more about allergies in a book called *Allergies and Children* by Milton Gold and Barry Zimmerman (Cambridge University Press).

ANAPHYLACTIC SHOCK

This is the name of a massive allergic reaction to a substance that gets into the child's body. The substance could be an injection (even one especially for children, such as immunisation) or an insect sting (see also 'Stings' in Chapter 22 on Minor Injuries and Ilnesses) and it can also be a food to which the child is allergic. It usually develops after only a few seconds and is a medical emergency.

Occasionally this can happen after the child has taken penicillin, if you didn't know beforehand that he was allergic to it. At the first suspicious sign STOP THE MEDICINE *immediately* – even though the doctor may have told you to continue with it until the end of the course. Check with your doctor before starting the medicine again.

There may be other things including some foods to which the child is allergic that you may also not know about, but in these instances the re-action is slower and sometimes less severe (see above).

WHAT TO LOOK FOR

● A few seconds after the injection (or sting or food) the child will develop all the signs of shock (see Chapter 27 on Shock).

REMEMBER – SHOCK LOOKS LIKE THIS

- His face may be very pale and grey-looking
- His skin may feel cold and clammy
- His pulse may feel fast and weak
- He may be frightened and fidgety
- He may be very thirsty
- He may yawn and 'gasp' for air
- He may say everything feels fuzzy
- He may become unconscious

- He may say he feels sick or may actually vomit.
- He may find it difficult to breathe, and may wheeze or gasp for air.
- He may have a sneezing attack.
- He may start to itch and his skin may become bright red.
- His face may start to swell up, particularly around the eyes, and he may develop large red blotches, called urticaria, on his skin.
- His pulse will be rapid and weak.
- The child might lose consciousness.

WHAT TO DO

This is an absolute emergency.

- *You must get the child to hospital as quickly as possible.* Dial 999 for an ambulance and tell them exactly what has happened.

- If he is still conscious, talk to him calmly, tell him a doctor is coming, and that you want him to lie down (as this is the position that will help him most).

- If, however, he is having difficulty breathing, in spite of being in shock you must sit him up, unless he is feeling faint or wants to be sick, in which case put him in the Recovery Position. Try to make him as comfortable as possible but watch him carefully to make sure he is safe.

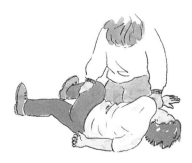

- If he becomes unconscious open his airway and check his breathing. If it stops, start your ABC Resuscitation Routine immediately until the ambulance arrives. A Paramedic is on most ambulances and he or she will be able to give your child the life-saving drugs he needs.

49

> **A** for **AIRWAY**   (is it clear?)
>
> **B** for **BREATHING**   (is he breathing?)
>
> **C** for **CIRCULATION**   (is his heart beating?)

There has recently been a slight increase in the number of children dying from allergic attacks. This is worrying doctors who specialise in childhood allergies and many feel that parents should have the medicine the child needs at home, rather than having to wait for a doctor or Paramedic to bring it.

If you would feel more comfortable learning how to use a pack like this, why don't you go and talk to your doctor about it. Or talk to the newly formed British Allergy Foundation (see page 47 for their address).

Remember, if your child is seriously allergic to a substance, penicillin for instance, he should wear a special bracelet (like Medic-Alert) saying so.

IF YOUR CHILD HAS A SEVERE ALLERGIC REACTION OR ANAPHYLACTIC SHOCK

- Calm him as much as possible. Tell him what you are doing.
- GET HELP URGENTLY. Call for an ambulance by dialling 999.
- Keep his airway as clear as possible. Sit him up on pillows with his arms resting on a table or cushions *or whatever position is most comfortable*.
- If he feels sick, lie him down and roll him into the Recovery Position, unless this distresses him more, in which case just make him safe and comfortable.

THINK

- Have you got help? Try shouting out of the window or front door.
- Have you called the ambulance? Try to get someone to do this for you.
- Shake and shout to the child to see if he is conscious.

IF THE CHILD BECOMES UNCONSCIOUS: be ready to start your ABC RESUSCITATION ROUTINE.

Now check   'A' for AIRWAY – is it clear?

IF HE DOESN'T RESPOND: OPEN THE AIRWAY. Tilt the child's head back and lift his chin forward. REMEMBER babies' necks are chubbier and more fragile. **Be gentle yet firm enough to tilt head back so airway is open.**

Now check   'B' for BREATHING

LOOK
LISTEN } for breathing
FEEL

IF THE CHILD IS NOT BREATHING: BREATHE FOR THE CHILD. Cover his mouth, or nose and mouth, with your mouth. Give him FIVE separate breaths. Watch his chest rise with each breath. *Less* breath for babies.

Now check   'C' for CIRCULATION

Is his heart beating? Check for the pulse. Feel the neck (or arm in a baby) for a pulse. **If there is no pulse and you haven't got help GET IT NOW.**

IF YOU CANNOT FEEL A PULSE: DO CHEST COMPRESSION. Feel for the right place – one finger-breadth below the nipple line. Press on the chest, at a rate of **100 presses per minute.**

For children over one year old: Use the 'heel' of one hand only, with your arm straight. **Press fifteen times to every two breaths** (so your hand presses in about 2.5-3.5cm or 1-1½ inches each time).

For babies: Use two fingers only and **press five times to one breath** (so your fingers press in about 2cm or about ¾ of an inch, each time).

KEEP DOING THIS UNTIL THE AMBULANCE ARRIVES.

5 ASTHMA

Twenty-five per cent of all children will suffer at least one asthmatic or wheezy attack by the time they are sixteen. Most of them develop the first symptoms during their primary school years, from the age of five to eleven. It is twice as common in boys as in girls.

What doctors now know is that if they treat children with 'wheezy' symptoms early enough they don't suffer as much as when they are left until they literally cannot breathe.

WHAT IS ASTHMA?

In asthma the muscles of the air passages go into spasm and tighten the airway. This usually happens in response to an allergic reaction of some kind, which varies from child to child. As the airway gets smaller it takes more and more effort to breathe air in and out, particularly breathing out. It feels like trying to take breaths through a small straw.

So you can understand why children might panic when they feel an attack coming on; and panic makes it worse. Don't ever let anyone persuade you that your child's asthma is 'only in the mind'. It isn't. It is a real disease, with real symptoms, and can cause a lot of real distress.

Why do children get asthma?

No one knows why children get asthma. A child may have more chance of getting it if someone in the family already has it. There are, however, 'triggers' to attacks which will affect one child more than another. You need to know about these since you may be able to prevent an attack, or at least lessen the effect of it, by giving the child his inhaler before or around the time he starts to wheeze or comes into contact with the 'trigger'. Alternatively you can keep him away from whatever it is that seems to cause an attack, although this is not always possible.

These are some of the 'triggers' that may affect children who get asthma:

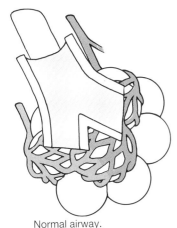

Normal airway.

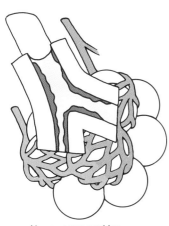

Airway narrowed by muscle spasm.

- *Infections* – usually a cold or flu, can often start a wheezy attack.

- *Allergies* – to feathers, house dust, animal hairs, pollen or anything that your child's body takes objection to. Don't keep a dog, cat or bird, for instance, if you feel there is even the slightest chance your child might be allergic to it.

- *Exercise* – particularly in cold, damp weather – tempting for your child to use as an excuse to miss PE!

- *Excitement* – either good or bad, such as fear or anger.

- *Air pollution* – such as cigarettes, aerosol sprays, bonfire smoke or car exhaust. When air pollution levels are high it will be reported on the national television weather forecasts.

- *Seasonal changes* – for instance when the pollen count goes up in the summer, the incidence of hay fever goes up too; or when it is suddenly very cold in winter. Pollen counts are often reported on weather bulletins.

- *Diet* – Allergies to food affect a very small number of children. If your child is allergic to a particular food he – and you – will know about it quite quickly because the effect is usually dramatic. It could be a response to a colouring material or preservative – so be aware. Lots of fresh fruit and raw vegetables are best.

The number of child deaths from asthma is quite high and is increasing. In 1991 there were sixteen deaths in children up to four years old; twenty-five in children from five to fourteen and *ninety* in children aged between fourteen to seventeen (it may be difficult to persuade your teenager to take his inhaler with him everywhere – he may not want to take a puff in front of his friends – but this is a real danger as you can see from the figures). Asthma is the commonest medical emergency in children but there is still very little information and education for parents, teachers and the children themselves. This may be because doctors do not recognise the warning signs early enough; or because parents don't give doctors the full picture – often because they genuinely don't understand the importance of doing so. And again some doctors are too laid back – perhaps they feel their asthma patients should stay calm – and fail to stress to parents the importance of recognising, and acting on, the first warning signs.

WHAT TO LOOK FOR

- These warning signs usually follow a pattern – a child might say, for example, that his chest feels tight, others may say something different – you know your child best.

- Most asthmatic children COUGH AT NIGHT. *This is one of the main things to look out for.* This can be very disturbing for a child – as well as for the poor parents – and it is hardly surprising therefore that children who cough instead of sleeping go through periods when they don't do well at school.

If you are worried about your child, take him to the doctor who will almost certainly listen to his chest and test how strongly he can blow through a 'peak flow meter'. This is a tube (a little smaller than an empty toilet roll) with a lip at the top, through which your child will blow. It measures how healthy your child's lungs are. If an asthmatic child is having a really bad time he will find it difficult to blow at all.

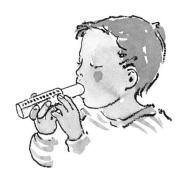

If the doctor thinks your child is asthmatic he will give him some medicine to breathe in through an inhaler when he has a wheezy attack, OR TO PREVENT ONE HAPPENING. The doctor will know which drugs your child will need.

There are two types of drug that can be given to an asthmatic child. These are classed by the National Asthma Campaign as Relievers and Preventers. The Preventers may be taken by the child every day to prevent an attack happening; they will keep down inflammation in the lungs. The Relievers give immediate relief by opening up the narrowed airways and allowing more air through into the lungs when an attack is already underway. They may also reduce redness and soreness of the air passages.

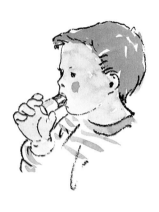

There are other ways of giving these drugs which your doctor might think will suit your child. He could give him a 'puffer', which works in a similar way to an inhaler; or tablets to take, either instead of or as well as inhaling.

If a child is a long-distance runner or plays a hefty game of rugger, particularly in damp weather, and knows that these activities may trigger an attack, then taking his medicine beforehand should protect him. But try to follow your doctor's advice on this. If you, or your child, don't think the inhaler is working, discuss this with your doctor. DON'T WAIT – it's important that you tackle any problems before they get out of hand.

If you or the doctor think your child is allergic to something in particular, he may suggest seeing a hospital Consultant specialising in allergies and asthma in children. This specialist doctor may do simple skin tests for allergic reactions. However, some doctors are not in favour of these tests because they feel a skin reaction may not give a true picture of how that same substance would react in the lungs.

In a skin test the doctor will put dots of 'substances' along the inside of one of the child's arms. This is to find out if the child is or is not allergic to a variety of things such as dog hairs, pollen, eggs, nuts and so on. He makes a pinprick through each dot to allow a small amount of the substance to enter the body. There will be a reaction on the skin if the child is allergic to it. It is useful for you to know if there is one particular thing to which the child is allergic.

Smoke irritates the lungs of healthy children, but for an asthmatic child it can really tip the balance between his being fairly well or being ill. If you are a smoker, try not to smoke near this child. Give it up if you can.

WHAT TO DO

If you (or your child) think he is getting an attack of asthma

- Reassure and calm him. This is basic but most important. If he starts to get nervous or to panic, it can make the attack worse. If you yourself are anxious, everything seems to tighten up inside. You may get a tummy ache or a headache, you may hunch your shoulders or start breathing faster. Imagine all this is on top of not being able to get your breath.

- Offer him a drink of water or a hot drink and suggest he moves to a different place if it will help him to feel more comfortable.

- Give him the inhaler or whatever medicine your doctor has given him.

- Try to make him rest. Do something with him that will take his mind off what is happening. You will know what works best, a favourite story or a game, or even watching television.

If the wheezing gets worse, or if he or you feel the inhaler (or medicine) is not working after two doses

- Call for the doctor immediately and explain clearly why you are calling. It is important that he understands the urgency of your call. Try not to let your child see how you are feeling.

- Reassure the child all the time. If he is small and feels he doesn't want to cuddle you (it might make him feel even more 'closed in' and panicky), give him a favourite teddy or toy instead. This may be difficult to get right – but be aware that whatever you get for him mustn't make him feel worse. Remember some toys may be very dusty (a teddy for instance) and if he is allergic to house dust – and the chances are he is – this could make him feel worse.

- REMEMBER panicking can only make the situation worse. You must resort to all the tricks you can to calm him.

If the attack gets worse, he cannot get his breath and his colour is poor

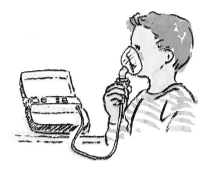

- Call for an ambulance by dialling 999. Tell the emergency operator what is happening. Some ambulance drivers are also Paramedics, which means they may be able to give drugs, and they will almost certainly carry a nebuliser on board. This is a special spray which the child puts over his face through a mask. It helps him to take up to ten times the normal dose of the drug he has in his inhaler. This will help him to breathe more easily by opening up his breathing passages.

- Reassure and calm him all the time.

55

● Encourage him to sit leaning slightly forward, resting on a table or some cushions. This is usually the best position in many situations where breathing is difficult.

● If the child becomes unconscious open his airway and check his breathing. If it stops, you must start your ABC Resuscitation Routine.

> **A** for **AIRWAY**   (is it clear?)
>
> **B** for **BREATHING**   (is he breathing?)
>
> **C** for **CIRCULATION**   (is his heart beating?)

Once the child gets to hospital he will be 'nebulised', if he hasn't been already. If he is having great difficulty breathing he will be given oxygen through a face mask and may also be given some drugs intravenously (by a needle into the vein). These will be stronger doses of the drugs he normally takes through his inhaler. They will help to reduce the redness and soreness of his air passages and widen them to help the air get through to the lungs more easily.

Occasionally a child may be put on a 'drip', which is a bottle of fluid which literally drips through a tube into the vein. This will be given if the child is in a severe state of shock.

If your child has asthma attacks and someone else looks after him

If you work full- or part-time and someone else looks after your child, it is important to tell them not only what medicine he takes and how he takes it, but also what will distract him once he feels an attack coming on. They must also be advised what to do in an emergency.

Asthma at school

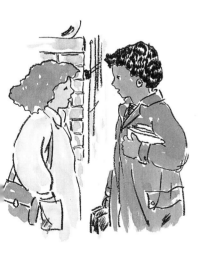

Teachers must be told, in a calm way, what happens if the child feels an attack coming. Some teachers are alarmed by children with asthma, while others can be stuck with old-fashioned ideas that 'it is all due to nerves', or 'he mustn't play games'. Some, on the other hand, are just brilliant and have exactly the right approach, being neither too sympathetic nor too stern, so the children *feel* their teachers understand and in turn feel they are safe. After all, can there BE anything worse than not being able to breathe properly?

If there is one thing guaranteed to make a child with asthma worse during his attack, it is thinking that he may not be able to get to the medicine he needs *when he needs it*.

If a child feels an attack coming on, and then has to start searching all over the school to find the teacher who has the key to the medicine cupboard (or medical room) so that he can use his inhaler, it is clearly going to make an unpleasant situation very much worse.

Most schools have rules about medicines being locked up and in the charge of one person. This obviously lessens the chances of a child overdosing with medicines which could be harmful, but asthmatic children should not suffer unnecessarily in the process. The important thing is for the child to be able to get to his inhaler quickly and with as little fuss as possible.

Having said that, children with asthma CAN play games, and take part in all activities if they want to. Teachers should not feel they must stop a child joining in anything – as long as the child feels all right about it and has used his inhaler if he needs to do so.

If you want further information contact:

National Asthma Campaign
Providence House, Providence Place, London N1 0NT.

Asthma Helpline 0345 010203
Ring between 1 p.m. and 9 p.m. (charged at local rate).

Or you may like to read *Childhood Asthma* by Neil Buchanan (Judy Piatkus Publishers Ltd), which answers many common questions parents have about asthma.

- Reassure and comfort the child.
- If he has an inhaler, tell him firmly but gently to use it.
- Sit him forward with a table or cushions in front of him so that he can rest on them.
- Call for an ambulance by dialling 999 – tell them what has happened.

THINK

- Have you managed to get some help? Try shouting out of the window or front door.
- Have you called for the ambulance? Try to get someone to do this for you.
- Have you checked for DANGER?
- Shake and shout to the child to see if he is conscious.

IF THE CHILD BECOMES UNCONSCIOUS: be ready to start your ABC RESUSCITATION ROUTINE.

Now check   'A' for AIRWAY – is it clear?

IF HE DOESN'T RESPOND: OPEN THE AIRWAY. Tilt the child's head back and lift his chin forward.

Now check   'B' for BREATHING

LOOK
LISTEN } for breathing
FEEL

IF THE CHILD IS NOT BREATHING: BREATHE FOR THE CHILD. Cover his mouth, or nose and mouth, with your mouth. Give him FIVE separate breaths. Watch his chest rise with each breath.

Now check   'C' for CIRCULATION

Is his heart beating? Feel the neck for a pulse. **If there is no pulse and you haven't got help GET IT NOW.**

IF YOU CANNOT FEEL A PULSE: DO CHEST COMPRESSION. Feel for the right place – one finger-breadth below the nipple line. Press on the chest, at a rate of **100 presses per minute.**

Use the 'heel' of one hand only, with your arm straight. **Press fifteen times to every two breaths** (so your hand presses in about 2.5-3.5cm or 1-1½ inches each time).

KEEP DOING THIS UNTIL THE AMBULANCE ARRIVES.

BLEEDING

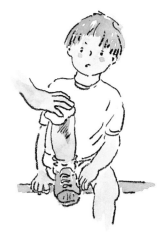

6

When a child cuts or grazes herself she bleeds, because the pressure in the blood vessels forces the blood out through this new 'opening' (the cut) in the skin.

If it is a graze the tiny amount of blood around the wound clots. It is a good idea to wash any wound like this gently with cool water, particularly if it is very dirty. It will then usually heal by itself.

Cover all cuts and grazes that are bleeding or oozing with a sticky plaster, and then as soon as healing has begun (usually about a day in children) take it off and let the air get to the wound. A plaster can be comforting, especially if it goes with a cuddle. Waterproof plasters tend to make the skin sweat and the cut may not heal as quickly as it should.

SEVERE BLEEDING

In a child ANY blood that flows from a vein or spurts out from an artery in a wound for longer than a few seconds is serious and if it is not treated URGENTLY the child could die (see Chapter 2 on How the Body Works). You must try to stop the bleeding as quickly as you can and call for medical help.

The dangers of losing a lot of blood

A child's body holds much less blood than an adult's. An adult can fairly 'comfortably' lose a pint of blood and will replace it quite quickly. But if a child loses the same amount it could be as much as a third or even *half* of her total amount of blood and it may be too much for her to cope with losing safely.

WHAT TO LOOK FOR

A child who loses a lot of blood will be in shock and may show all or some of the following reactions:

- Her face and lips will become pale and her skin will feel cool and clammy. She may be shivering.

- Her pulse will feel faster and weaker than normal because the heart has to work harder to pump less blood around the body.

- The child may feel frightened and fidgety – an older child may be unusually talkative and restless.

- She may be very thirsty. This is the body's natural urge to put back the fluid that has been lost.

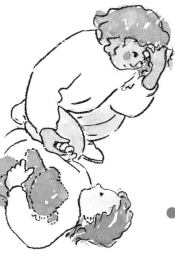

- She may 'gasp' for air. This also is a natural bodily response to try to replace the oxygen that has been lost in the blood.

- She may tell you that everything feels 'fuzzy' or she may not seem to know where she is or what has happened to her. If she is standing up, she may faint.

Bleeding is frightening, both to the injured child and to the adult who is trying to help. Some people feel faint at the sight of blood. If you tend to do this, don't worry; if it is your child and you are the only one around to give first aid, your adrenalin (the body's natural 'buzz' chemical for fight or flight) will carry you through, and the chances of your fainting are very slight.

WHAT TO DO

- If the child loses consciousness you must check to see if she is breathing. If not start your ABC Resuscitation Routine immediately.

> **A** for **AIRWAY**   (is it clear?)
>
> **B** for **BREATHING**   (is she breathing?)
>
> **C** for **CIRCULATION**   (is her heart beating?)

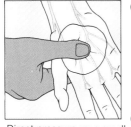

Direct pressure on a small wound.

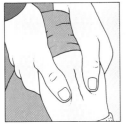

If it's a large gash, press around the sides.

- If she remains unconscious but is breathing and you feel she could be sick – she might be making choking noises – roll her gently into the Recovery Position *before you start looking after her injury*. Otherwise if you leave her on her back you might be so busy stopping the bleeding that you don't notice her vomit, and this may block the airway and stop her breathing.

- Once you are sure her breathing is all right, then attend to the wound AS QUICKLY AS YOU CAN. The quicker you can stop the bleeding the less chance there is of shock developing.

- If blood is pumping out of a wound all you can do is to press on the wound to stop the bleeding. This is called 'direct pressure'. DO NOT start poking the wound – it will make the bleeding worse. If possible you should use a clean pad to press on the wound. However, the most important thing is to stop the bleeding, so if you don't have one use your bare hands or the pads of your fingers. You may have to squeeze the edges of the wound together if the sides are gaping. Press around the sides, as you do so, rather than on top. If you use a dressing it should be *larger* on all sides than the wound.

60

- DO NOT REMOVE ANYTHING from a deep wound. It might be like the cork in a bottle – as soon as you pull it out you will open up the blood vessel and the bleeding may be much more difficult, if not impossible, to control.

- Bandage the dressing in place. Tie it firmly enough to control the bleeding, but not so tight that it cuts off the circulation completely. If the child has hurt an arm or a leg, look at her fingers or toes nearest the dressing at frequent intervals. If it is too tight they will begin to look blue, in which case you must loosen the dressing right away. If the child is able to speak she may tell you they feel 'tingly'. If the wound starts to bleed again because you have loosened the bandage too much, really press hard directly on the wound itself (as well as putting on a firm but slightly looser dressing).

- Keep pressing on the wound for about fifteen to twenty minutes – enough time to allow the blood vessels to narrow, for the blood to clot and if necessary for medical help to arrive.

- If a lot of blood keeps coming through the bandage DO NOT REMOVE IT. Simply *put another bandage on top* of the first one.

- Lie the child down and raise the injured part as high as you can above the level of the heart. This helps to lessen the pressure and slow down the amount of blood coming out of the wound. But if the child has gashed her head, gently prop her up on pillows or cushions.

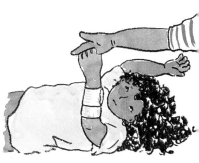

- Call for the ambulance by dialling 999, if you haven't been able to do so up to now. Tell them what has happened.

- Don't forget to reassure the child and tell her that everything will be all right.

- WASH YOUR HANDS with soap and water after handling blood, even if it is your own child's.

The sight of a lot of blood can be frightening to anyone, but particularly to a small child. Remember though, blood loss often looks worse than it really is. If it is possible, find a favourite teddy or doll for the child to cuddle; she may be too badly hurt or in pain to have a cuddle from you and something familiar can be comforting and reassuring.

All children with SERIOUS WOUNDS must go to hospital.

If you are unable to stop the bleeding

- You will need expert medical help quickly. Tell her that you are going to call an ambulance and dial 999. If you have to leave the child for a moment to do this, then you must make sure that her airway is clear. If you can, put her in the Recovery Position – especially if she is too badly injured to carry with you to the phone. Tell the Ambulance Service exactly what has happened or as much as you know, and that you cannot stop the bleeding.

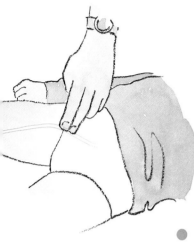

● If you haven't a phone *stand on the front doorstep and shout for help*. Make sure that someone calls for an ambulance.

● When there are a lot of serious wounds on one limb you probably won't be able to treat them all at once, so apply INDIRECT PRESSURE to the *main artery* of that limb. This is the main stop-cock, if you like, for that particular limb and is the quickest way to stop the bleeding in these sorts of multiple injuries. The main arteries are to be found against the bones. (See Chapter 2 on How the Body Works.) You may have to press on the artery very hard indeed to stop the bleeding, but do not apply indirect pressure *for longer than ten minutes* – it cuts off the blood supply to the limb. If you continue to hold that position, the blood supply could be permanently cut off and the arm or leg damaged so much that the child could lose the limb. In an emergency, however, if there is no other way to stop the bleeding, it may be all you can do – and it could save the child's life.

If there is something stuck in the wound

● You wouldn't be able to wash it away – DO NOT remove it.

● Reassure her and explain what you are going to do.

● Apply pressure *around* the wound, rather than directly on to it. You do this by squeezing the edges of the cut together, keeping the thing that is sticking out in the centre. If it is glass, you have to be particularly careful, so that you don't cause any further injury.

● If it is a bone that is sticking up through the skin, treat it in the same way but try to stop the child from moving it. This needs to be explained to her if she is old enough to understand (see Chapter 18 on Fractures and Bone Injuries).

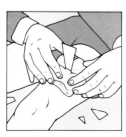

● Use two clean pads to hold the edges of the wound together, or the cleanest thing you have to hand. Build up whatever padding you have carefully around the sides of the object, so that it is well protected and can't do any more damage.

● Bandage firmly in position, if possible using a criss-cross movement *around the padding only*, although this is a bit tricky. Whatever you do DON'T BANDAGE OVER THE TOP of the sticking-out object – this will press it further into the wound.

● Raise the limb so that it is higher than the heart. If the child has cut her head and there is something sticking in the wound, sit her up.

● If you haven't already done so, call the ambulance by dialling 999.

● Watch for signs of shock and REMEMBER pain increases the chance of shock, so try not to cause unnecessary pain while you are dealing with the injury.

REMEMBER – SHOCK LOOKS LIKE THIS

- Her face may be very pale and grey-looking
- Her skin may feel cold and clammy
- Her pulse may feel fast and weak
- She may be frightened and fidgety
- She may be very thirsty
- She may yawn and 'gasp' for air
- She may say everything feels fuzzy
- She may become unconscious

- Once you have stemmed the bleeding and have called the ambulance, the best thing you can do is to sit and hold her and talk to her. She may not respond much, but she will be reassured by your voice. If you still have to rush around and can't sit with her, give her her favourite teddy or doll to cuddle – it's the next best thing.

- DO NOT give her anything to eat or drink in case she has to have an anaesthetic.

- REMEMBER if the child loses consciousness you must check her breathing. If it stops, start your ABC Resuscitation Routine *before you do anything else*.

A for **AIRWAY**   (is it clear?)

B for **BREATHING**   (is she breathing?)

C for **CIRCULATION**   (is her heart beating?)

Once you are satisfied that she is breathing normally again, carry on treating the wound.

- If you think the child might be sick, either turn her into the Recovery Position or, if she is too badly injured to move her, turn her head to one side, so that if she is sick there is less danger of her inhaling it and blocking her airway.

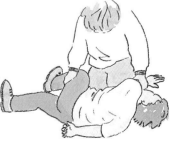

LUNGS

After a 'crush' injury to the chest, a child may cough up pink, frothy blood from her lungs. She will have serious breathing problems and will be frightened, agitated and in great pain.

You will hear a 'sucking' sound. This means that the chest wall has been punctured and air is getting into the lung space; there may also be blood bubbling from this wound as the child breathes out.

The more air that gets into the chest cavity the more the lung collapses (the lung itself may also be damaged), and the child will become very short of oxygen. However, *do not attempt to seal off the wound*, as this could make the situation worse.

WHAT TO DO

This is an ABSOLUTE MEDICAL EMERGENCY and one of the most frightening accidents that can happen to a child. She needs to be calmed as much as possible. The calmer she is the quieter her breathing will become, and the more oxygen there will be for her. So RE-ASSURE HER a lot and tell her what you are going to do.

- You must GET HELP QUICKLY. Phone for an ambulance by dialling 999. *Don't wait – it won't get better on its own.* Tell them what has happened. If you haven't got a phone stand on the front doorstep and shout for help.

- Gently prop up the child on pillows or cushions, to help her breathe more easily, *leaning her towards the injured side.*

- Put a pillow gently under her legs to lessen any tension on the chest, and also to reduce shock.

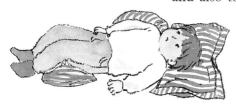

- REMEMBER if the child loses consciousness you must check her breathing and if it stops, start your ABC Resuscitation Routine immediately.

> **A** for **AIRWAY**   (is it clear?)
>
> **B** for **BREATHING**   (is she breathing?)
>
> **C** for **CIRCULATION**   (is her heart beating?)

ABDOMEN

A child may bleed from or into her tummy area.

If a child has a bad abdominal (tummy) wound, bleeding could be happening outside *and* inside her body – a part of her intestines may be sticking out through the wound. This is a very dangerous situation, not only because of shock due to the loss of blood, but because the internal organs could become infected if they are exposed to the germs in the air.

WHAT TO LOOK FOR

- One of the main signs may be shock, which you often get with internal bleeding (see Chapter 27 on Shock).

REMEMBER – SHOCK LOOKS LIKE THIS

- Her face may be very pale and grey-looking

- Her skin may feel cold and clammy

- Her pulse may feel fast and weak

- She may be frightened and fidgety

- She may be very thirsty

- She may yawn and 'gasp' for air

- She may say everything feels fuzzy

- She may become unconscious

- There may be only a small puncture wound on the outside of the body, or there may be a gash – with or without the intestines poking through. Both are serious injuries.

- She may be sick, and will certainly be in a lot of pain.

WHAT TO DO

- Lie the child gently on the floor and slide a pillow under her bent knees to support them. This will help to take the very painful pressure off her tummy.

- Put a sterile (if possible) or clean dressing over the wound as gently as possible and keep it in place with a bandage or plaster. Make sure the dressing is larger than the wound. *Do this, even though there may be some intestines sticking out.* The important thing is to cover them quickly to

65

prevent infection from getting in. DO NOT use sticky or fluffy dressings – a plastic bag is as good as anything.

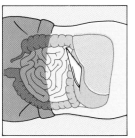

- DO NOT remove anything that may be sticking out of the wound. If you think you can see something sharp, cover it lightly with a piece of sterile or clean gauze – or the cleanest thing you can find, such as a recently ironed handkerchief. Then gently pack something clean (dressings if possible) around the object to prevent it from moving and doing further damage. Bandage around the *sides of the wound only*. Don't squash the intestines – they are very delicate and you may damage them.

- The child may want to vomit, so you must support her tummy by pressing gently on the dressing. This is to prevent the internal organs from coming out – or to stop those already poking out from escaping any further with the force of the vomiting. (Sneezing or coughing would have the same effect.)

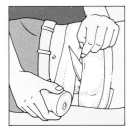

- If her injury will allow it, roll her gently onto her side, *away from the wound*, into the Recovery Position, supporting her tummy as you do so. If she is too badly injured to move but is fully conscious, turn her head to one side so that if she does vomit she will be less likely to inhale it and block her airway.

- This is a very frightening and painful injury and she will need lots of reassurance and comfort. Talk to her all the time you are looking after her and tell her what you are going to do, even though you may feel that she is too ill to take much notice – the sound of your voice will be comforting.

- If she becomes unconscious you must watch her breathing and if it stops, start your ABC Resuscitation Routine right away.

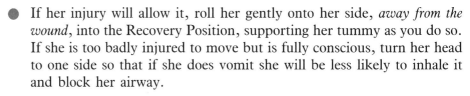

A for **AIRWAY**   (is it clear?)

B for **BREATHING**   (is she breathing?)

C for **CIRCULATION**   (is her heart beating?)

- This child needs urgent medical attention. If you haven't already done so, call for an ambulance by dialling 999. Tell them the sort of injuries that she has and what you have done.

AMPUTATIONS

If the child cuts herself so badly that the limb, finger or toe is cut off completely, you have two alternatives. If you can, be super-cool and stop the bleeding, as described above, then pick up the amputated bit, wrap it up in something clean – or better still put it in a plastic bag surrounded by ice if possible – and label it with your child's name and the time the accident happened. (The child then has a good chance of having it sewn back on again. Micro-surgery has made huge advances in this field. *But the child and the part that has been cut off must arrive at the hospital at the same time.*)

Or you may decide that this is too much for you, and just deal with the child's injury. Unfortunately there is no other way of replacing a limb at present. You can only do what you feel you can do.

Everyone hopes these things won't happen, but they do, and if you understand what you might have to do, it may help you to make some pretty important decisions.

If the limb, fingers or toes are crushed, put a clean dressing on the wounds and bandage firmly to stop the bleeding. Get the child to hospital as soon as you can. Tips of fingers trapped in doors will be soothed by holding them under cold water until the pain eases. Paracetamol-syrup might also help if she is in a lot of pain. Get the hospital to relieve the pressure from a blood clot under the finger nail by piercing the finger nail. It sounds awful but it gives tremendous relief.

INTERNAL BLEEDING

Of course, bleeding doesn't only happen on the outside of the body. After any injury that involves bones breaking or the body being crushed in some way – say by a car, or a heavy object falling onto the child, or by being hit or shaken hard – the internal organs can be damaged so much that they bleed inside the body (see Chapter 2 on How the Body Works).

Internal bleeding can be more serious than bleeding that you can see, because it is often difficult to recognise. There may be tell-tale signs like bruising on the skin, but otherwise there may be no evidence of what is happening *inside* the child's body.

If the escaping blood oozes into a cavity like the chest or the skull, it can do a lot of damage by pressing on the lung, the brain or whatever vital organ is in that particular space. It also cuts down the amount of blood going round the child's body, causing her blood pressure to fall (see Chapter 2 on How the Body Works).

Internal bleeding can be very painful and causes severe shock but often shows no signs at all for some time.

ALWAYS SUSPECT INTERNAL BLEEDING AFTER A VIOLENT INJURY, especially if there are signs of shock and you can't see any blood. Watch the child carefully if you think this may have happened.

67

WHAT TO LOOK FOR

- What was the child doing immediately before she became ill?

- The child may be in severe pain, and there might also be swelling and local tenderness, in her tummy, for instance.

- She will become restless and show signs and symptoms of shock such as yawning and gasping for air, because of the loss of oxygen in her blood. She may be thirsty because of the amount of fluid she is losing (see Chapter 27 on Shock).

REMEMBER – SHOCK LOOKS LIKE THIS

- Her face may be very pale and grey-looking

- Her skin may feel cold and clammy

- Her pulse may feel fast and weak

- She may be frightened and fidgety

- She may be very thirsty

- She may yawn and 'gasp' for air

- She may say everything feels fuzzy

- She may become unconscious

- *Blood may appear from any opening in the child's body.*

WHAT TO DO

There is very little first aid you can give for internal bleeding. All you can do is to put the child in the most comfortable position.

- If you think she is bleeding from the abdomen, it may help to put a cushion or pillow under her head and another under her knees. This will relieve some of the tension on her tummy. Comfort and reassure her a lot and get her to hospital as quickly as possible.

- She needs immediate medical attention. Don't wait if you think she may have internal bleeding. Call an ambulance by dialling 999 and tell them what has happened.

- If the child becomes unconscious watch her breathing carefully and if it stops, start your ABC Resuscitation Routine right away.

A for **AIRWAY**   (is it clear?)

B for **BREATHING**   (is she breathing?)

C for **CIRCULATION**   (is her heart beating?)

MOUTH

She may vomit blood from her stomach, although this is unusual in children.

This blood is sometimes described as 'coffee grounds' – if it is semi-digested blood – but it may also be bright red, depending on what is causing it. She may be bleeding from inside the mouth or throat, or she may have swallowed a small, sharp-edged toy which has cut her on the way to her tummy. If she has had her tonsils out recently, one of the tonsil-beds may be bleeding. All of these need urgent attention.

See also 'Teeth' in Chapter 22 on Minor Injuries and Illnesses.

WHAT TO DO

● Lie her down with her head to one side in the Recovery Position. If she has just had her tonsils out, raise her head and shoulders, still keeping her head on one side.

ANUS (or back-passage)

A child may pass blood in her motions, or just onto her pants. You need to make sure it is not coming from the vagina (see below).

If the child goes to the toilet and passes a black, 'tarry', smelly stool it might mean that she is bleeding from her upper bowel. If she passes fresh, bright-red blood it means that she is bleeding from the lower bowel or anus (back-passage).

Either of these could happen as a result of a violent injury or because of disease in the bowel. The child will almost certainly be in severe pain and there may also be swelling and local tenderness, for example in her tummy.

She might show signs and symptoms of shock such as yawning and gasping – because there is too little oxygen in the blood – and thirst because of the loss of fluid.

69

WHAT TO DO

- Put the child in the most comfortable position and treat for shock (see Chapter 27 on Shock).

> ### REMEMBER – SHOCK LOOKS LIKE THIS
> - Her face may be very pale and grey-looking
> - Her skin may feel cold and clammy
> - Her pulse may feel fast and weak
> - She may be frightened and fidgety
> - She may be very thirsty
> - She may yawn and 'gasp' for air
> - She may say everything feels fuzzy
> - She may become unconscious

- Reassure her a lot, talk to her and tell her what you are going to do.

- REMEMBER if the child loses consciousness you must check her breathing and if it stops, start your ABC Resuscitation Routine immediately.

> **A** for **AIRWAY** (is it clear?)
>
> **B** for **BREATHING** (is she breathing?)
>
> **C** for **CIRCULATION** (is her heart beating?)

- If you have not already done so, depending on the amount of pain, distress and shock she is in, either call her GP or get her to hospital urgently.

Bleeding from the anus could mean that the child has been sexually abused. If you suspect this has happened, there may be other signs to look out for (see Chapter 26 on Sexual Abuse).

VAGINA (front-passage)

The child may pass blood from her vagina. You need to make sure it is not coming from the anus (see above).

Your child may have started her periods – some girls start as early as eight or nine years of age. If, however, she is not coming up to puberty it could mean that she has a vaginal injury or she might have been sexually abused (see Chapter 26 on Sexual Abuse).

If she has started her periods there is a possibility that she could have been pregnant – in other words she may have miscarried. This may be difficult for you to think about.

WHAT TO DO

If she is in pain, or there is a lot of blood

● Lie her down and raise her legs and head. This will take any pressure off her tummy and make her feel a little better.

● Reassure the child. Blood is frightening and when it comes from 'down there' – when you're not used to it – it may seem to be worse than it is. (Even when you *are* used to it and it's at the wrong time or the wrong amount, it can be scary!)

● Call for an ambulance by dialling 999 and tell them what has happened (or at least as much as you know).

● Treat her for shock (see Chapter 27 on Shock).

> **REMEMBER – SHOCK LOOKS LIKE THIS**
> ● Her face may be very pale and grey-looking
> ● Her skin may feel cold and clammy
> ● Her pulse may feel fast and weak
> ● She may be frightened and fidgety
> ● She may be very thirsty
> ● She may yawn and 'gasp' for air
> ● She may say everything feels fuzzy
> ● She may become unconscious

If she is in no pain and there is only a little blood

Reassure her; whatever else, she will be anxious. If you think she has just begun her periods and you haven't told her about it, now is the time to do so. The first thing is to congratulate her on becoming a woman! The earlier you start to talk about this the better, but if you feel uncomfortable talking to her about it – and some people do – there are some really good books on the subject, for example *Have You Started Yet?* by Ruth Thomson; and *The Body Book* by Claire Rayner, which deals with all sorts of things to do with our bodies and not only periods. (It is better for her and for you if she is prepared well in advance.)

Bleeding from the vagina in a child or young girl is not normal (apart from periods). You need to know if she has injured herself in some way or if someone (or something) has injured her. We know a girl who split her vagina coming down a water chute, as she hit the water at speed in the local swimming baths. This is a typical 'water-skiing' injury.

If you have a sympathetic GP you may want to talk to him (or her) about it, preferably with your child. Don't forget that if you normally see a male doctor and there is a female doctor in the practice, they may allow you to see her if you explain that you (or your daughter) would find it easier.

If you are not sure why she is bleeding, get her medical help at hospital.

URETHRA

The child may pass blood through the urethra (the tube joining the bladder to the outside) which will appear in the urine.

This is usually smoky-coloured, or she/he may pass bright-red blood. Either may mean that there is some injury, or disease to the bladder, kidneys, vagina or penis. If your child is not in pain, see your GP first. But he almost certainly will be, so you will need to stress it is urgent.

A not uncommon injury for boys is to get their penis caught in their fly-zip; or they may poke something into their penis. As a staff-nurse in Casualty, I was often seeing boys admitted with knitting needles or other 'things' firmly stuck up the shaft of their penis. Whether he has pushed something into his penis or it has got caught in his zip, he will be equally distressed.

(If your child experiments in this way try not to be too annoyed with him. Most children explore their genitals in one way or another, some more than others. This is normal and it is better not to overreact, no matter how tempting it might be. He will be in great pain and will probably be in shock.)

WHAT TO DO

Lie the child down with his head and legs raised. This will take a lot of the pressure off his pelvic area (the bit around his penis). The child will be in pain and will probably be very anxious. Make sure he understands that you are not cross and try to comfort him as best you can. Tell him what you are going to do and reassure him that hospitals are used to dealing with things like this (because they are).

- Send for an ambulance by dialling 999 and explain exactly what has happened.

- Treat him for shock (see Chapter 27 on Shock).

REMEMBER – SHOCK LOOKS LIKE THIS

- His face may be very pale and grey-looking

- His skin may feel cold and clammy

- His pulse may feel fast and weak

- He may be frightened and fidgety

- He may be very thirsty

- He may yawn and 'gasp' for air

- He may say everything feels fuzzy

- He may become unconscious

NOSE

A child may bleed from the nose.

Nose-bleeds are common in children, particularly in hot weather. Although they are bloody and messy they are rarely serious and it is not usually necessary for the child to see a doctor.

You must, however, *call for medical help if*:

- The nose-bleed continues for over half an hour.

- The child has just had a bad fall or crack on the head.

- The blood is mixed with clear fluid. This might suggest that the child's skull is fractured (see Chapter 19 on Head Injuries).

WHAT TO DO

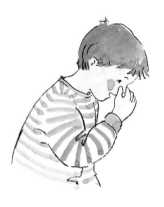

For a simple nose-bleed:

- Sit the child forward and let the blood drip away. Pinch the soft part of the nose above the nostrils – an older child can do this herself.

- If it is a bad nose-bleed, some crushed ice (or a few frozen peas in a plastic bag if you have no ice) placed on the bridge of the nose will help to cool and therefore clot the blood. This will help the nose-bleed to stop.

- In a bad nose-bleed keep pinching the top of the nose for ten minutes then check to see if it has stopped.

- Tell the child not to talk (impossible for some) and not to swallow, cough, sniff, or blow her nose.

- NEVER poke anything into the nose in an attempt to stop the bleeding – it will stop by itself.

Most children who have frequent nose-bleeds get used to them and can treat them themselves.

EAR

A child may bleed from inside the ear canal.

This usually means that the ear-drum has ruptured. More seriously it would show that the child has fractured her skull – particularly if the blood is mixed with clear fluid. You may suspect this if she has recently fallen or been knocked over.

WHAT TO DO

- Reassure the child. She will be frightened and almost certainly in pain. Talk to her calmly and gently and tell her what you are going to do.

- Lie the child down, but gently raise her head and shoulders with her head leaning over towards the injured ear so that any blood or fluid can drain out.

- Cover the ear with a sterile dressing or with the cleanest thing you can find. Bandage it very gently in position (see Chapter 19 on Head Injuries).

- This child needs to see a doctor URGENTLY. Call for an ambulance by dialling 999.

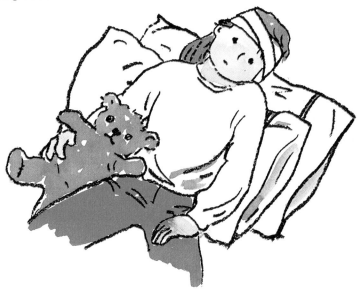

TEETH

A child may bleed from a tooth socket.

WHAT TO DO

This may be from a tooth that has been knocked out, or which has come out by itself, and bleeding will usually stop on its own – helped along by swilling the mouth out with cold water. You can add a pinch of salt to the water to cut down the risk of infection, but if the child can't bear the taste it is more important for her to rinse out with plain water.

If, however, the bleeding doesn't stop, then ask the child to 'bite' on a sterile or clean dressing – an eye-pad is ideal – and keep the pressure up for about ten minutes. If the bleeding does not stop by then she should see her dentist or a doctor.

Sit the child down quietly and encourage her to hold her head up. This position will lessen the oozing (see 'Teeth' in Chapter 22 on Minor Injuries and Illnesses).

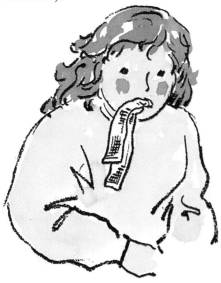

THINK

- Have you got help? Try shouting out of the window or front door.
- Have you called an ambulance? Get someone to do this.
- Have you checked for DANGER?
- Shake and shout to the child to see if she is conscious.

If she is breathing:
- Reassure and comfort the child. TREAT HER FOR SHOCK.
- Put direct pressure on the wound – if there is something stuck in it DO NOT remove it, but put pressure *around* the object.
- If a limb is bleeding, raise it above the level of the heart.
- Call for an ambulance. Dial 999. Tell them what has happened.
- If the child feels sick, roll her into the Recovery Position.

If she has a CHEST WOUND (crush injury)
- *Gently* prop her head on pillows, leaning her towards the injured side.

If she has INTERNAL BLEEDING – ABDOMEN
- If the area around her tummy is painful, put a pillow *gently* under her head and another under her knees.

IF THE CHILD BECOMES UNCONSCIOUS: be ready to start your ABC RESUSCITATION ROUTINE.

Now check   'A' for AIRWAY – is it clear?

OPEN THE AIRWAY. Tilt the child's head back and lift her chin forward. REMEMBER babies' necks are chubbier and more fragile.

Now check   'B' for BREATHING

LOOK
LISTEN } for breathing
FEEL

IF THE CHILD IS NOT BREATHING: BREATHE FOR THE CHILD. Cover her mouth, or nose and mouth, with your mouth. Give her FIVE separate breaths. Watch her chest rise with each breath (*less* breath for babies).

Now check   'C' for CIRCULATION

Is her heart beating? Feel the neck (or arm in a baby) for a pulse.

IF YOU CANNOT FEEL A PULSE: DO CHEST COMPRESSION. Feel for the right place – one finger-breadth below the nipple line. Press on the chest, at a rate of **100 presses per minute.**

For children over one year old: Use the 'heel' of one hand only, with your arm straight. **Press fifteen times to every two breaths** (so your hand presses in about 2.5-3.5cm or 1-1½ inches each time).

For babies: Use two fingers only and **press five times to one breath** (so your fingers press in about 2cm or about ¾ of an inch, each time).

KEEP DOING THIS UNTIL THE AMBULANCE ARRIVES.

BURNS AND SCALDS

7

Over 50,000 children, most of them under five years of age, go to hospital each year because of burning or scalding accidents. Many of these accidents could be avoided, and parents need to be aware of the danger zones, particularly in the home.

The difference between a burn and a scald is that burns are caused by a dry heat, and scalds are caused by something wet and very hot, such as liquid, oil or steam.

Chemicals, electric shocks and radiation (by over-exposure to the sun) can also cause burns. Extreme cold can 'burn' – so *don't* ask a small child to get something from the freezer unless you have explained to her that frozen food, *particularly in a metal container*, can burn in the same way as hot objects and should be carried with a cloth.

One thing that burns and scalds have in common is that they HURT – you only have to think of any small burn you may have had yourself, perhaps while cooking, to know the unexpected pain and distress it causes.

Watch microwave-heated fluids. You must stir them from time to time during cooking otherwise you will get 'hot-spot boil-overs'. This means that if you jog the cup the cold fluid knocks the hot, making it spill out unexpectedly. Likewise always break egg yolks before you microwave them. They have been known to explode and burn when taken out of the microwave.

Older children who run their own bath may forget the importance of running the cold water first. And when they help with the cooking, they may not realise how hot the mixture is becoming as they stir and splash.

If children injure themselves, it is IMPORTANT that you know how to give the right first aid treatment, quickly, quietly and with lots of reassurance to the child.

MINOR BURNS

Minor burns are smaller than a two-pence piece or exactly 1 inch or 2.5cm.

WHAT TO DO

- Gently place the burned area in a bowl of *cold water for at least* TEN MINUTES or more, or until the child says the pain is easing, then cover with a clean dry non-fluffy cloth kept in place with a bandage or a clean scarf.

- Use any bland, cold liquid such as milk or lemonade to bathe the area, if you cannot get to any water.

- If there is anything tight around the area that has been burned, such as a ring or bracelet, take it off quickly, so that it doesn't get trapped as the skin swells.

- DO NOT BREAK ANY BLISTERS or peel off any skin. All this may do is infect the burn, making it harder for it to heal without scarring.

- DO NOT put any lotions, potions, ointment or oils on the burn – no matter how tempted you might be by 'magic cure' stories. Just cover with the dry non-fluffy dressing and leave alone.

- DO NOT put any sort of sticking plaster on any but the smallest burns (less than the size of a two-pence piece), because if the skin is burned, you could peel off the skin when you peel off the plaster.

- ANY BURN OR SCALD THAT IS BIGGER THAN A TWO-PENCE PIECE (1 inch or 2.5cm) is considered to be a serious injury and SHOULD BE SEEN BY A DOCTOR, because there is *danger of infection and shock*.

FIRE ACCIDENTS

WHAT TO DO

- Lift or, if you have to, drag the child away from the heat; being as careful as possible not to burn yourself or set yourself alight in the process.

- If her clothing is on fire remember this: STOP, DROP and ROLL.

- STOP: Don't waste time looking for water to douse the flames (unless you happen to be near a large enough quantity of water in a bucket or a bath).

- DROP: Get the child down on the floor. This does two things: it stops the child from panicking and running round the room, therefore fanning the flames; it also stops the fire from rising up towards the child's face. Remember that heat and flames rise. If the bottom of her nightdress catches fire and the child is standing up, the flames will soon rise to her hair and face. (Think what happens when you hold a lighted match downwards, how quickly the flame comes up towards your fingers.)

- ROLL her *onto* the flames and smother them with a large, heavy piece of material – fireproof if possible (in other words, one which won't easily catch fire or melt). The Fire Brigade recommends using curtains (the heavier the better), if you can pull them off the rails and quickly wrap them round the child. Even if the material *could* catch fire they will probably stop the flames and prevent any more oxygen getting to the fire. This will stop further injury to the child.

● If there are any small flames licking around the sides of the material you can stamp them out with a heavy item of clothing such as a jacket, or, if you have to, with a hand or foot.

● Protect the child's face by pulling any burning clothing away from it.

● If the child has been splashed with burning fat or oil and you happen to be in the kitchen (where these sorts of accidents usually happen), you must move her away from the burning oil or fat pan and gently splash or pour cold water onto the child's skin.

● One way of cooling a burn is to find the inside of something clean that has recently been ironed and which is big enough to cover the burnt area. Put it straight onto the child's skin and splash cold water onto it. Keep doing this at regular intervals until the ambulance arrives.

● Do not in any circumstances put water ANYWHERE NEAR A BURNING OIL OR FAT PAN. Just turn off the heat – and if you have an electric cooker, remove the pan from the source of the heat – then cover it, either with a fire blanket or the lid of the pan. (Putting water on it would make the fire go completely out of control.)

It makes good sense to have a fire blanket handy in the kitchen, especially if you have children in the house. You just cover the burning pan with the cloth, move the pan from the heat and smother the flames. *Leave the cloth on top of the pan until it is cool.*

SEVERE BURNS

WHAT TO LOOK FOR

● However small the burn is, there will usually be severe pain in and around the injured part UNLESS the burn is so deep that it has destroyed the nerve endings in the skin, when the child won't feel the pain.

● There may be redness and swelling, although this may not happen immediately, but unless the burn is cooled quickly the skin will swell and then blister and peel.

● Alternatively the skin might look waxy and grey, or may even be charred and feel numb. This always means a deep burn.

● The child will almost certainly be in shock (see Chapter 27 on Shock).

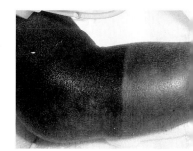

First degree burn. These are usually just red and sore areas – sunburn is included – but occasionally the skin will blister or swell.

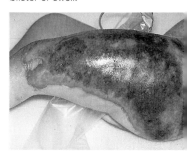

Second degree burn. This is much redder, more painful and the skin is blistered. The skin will usually heal, however, without scarring.

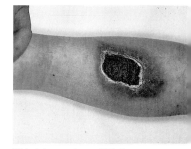

Third degree burn. This is the most severe burn and means that the whole layer of skin has been burnt off exposing the nerves. The child is in great pain.

REMEMBER – SHOCK LOOKS LIKE THIS

- Her face may be very pale and grey-looking
- Her skin may feel cold and clammy
- Her pulse may feel fast and weak
- She may be frightened and fidgety
- She may be very thirsty
- She may yawn and 'gasp' for air
- She may say everything feels fuzzy
- She may become unconscious

All severe burns (especially 'numb' burns) MUST BE SEEN URGENTLY BY A DOCTOR.

WHAT TO DO

- *Cool the area that has been burnt,* as quickly as possible, to prevent the heat of the burn spreading further outwards and downwards into the tissues. Cooling will also help to relieve the pain and lessen the chance of a shock (see below).

- Carefully pour jugs of cold water or any other cold, harmless, liquid such as milk if you are not near any water, over the burnt area. Keep doing this until the child tells you the pain is getting better – *but for at least ten minutes*. Once the clothes have cooled down, tell her that you are going to take them off her and then *gently* do this.

- NEVER REMOVE ANY CLOTHES THAT HAVE STUCK TO THE SKIN. If necessary, cut the unstuck clothes from around the burnt area – BUT DO NOT PULL as you can easily cause more injury and drag on the burnt flesh.

- ALWAYS reassure, comfort and explain what you are doing. I cannot stress the importance of this too much. Cuddle her if possible where she is not burnt or see if you can find her favourite teddy or doll and give it to her, making sure that it doesn't touch the burn.

- DO NOT give her anything to drink in case she has to go to the operating theatre when she gets to hospital. You can, if you like, just wet her mouth with a clean hanky or piece of gauze dipped in cold water. This might make her feel more comfortable.

- REMOVE ANY TIGHT CLOTHING and watches, bracelets, belts, necklets or rings from around the burn as soon as you can, otherwise the area will swell and these will be much more difficult and painful to remove later.

● COVER THE BURN QUICKLY, having cooled the burnt area first. If you only cover it, the burning process continues.

Skin protects the body from infection and when it is burnt, it allows fluid 'serum' to seep out into the tissues, and infection to get in, through the wound caused by the burn. This can set in very quickly so it is important that you cover the burn as soon as you can. This can be done ideally with a large pre-packed sterile dressing, but if not, with a clean, recently ironed, non-fluffy cloth – the inside of a sheet, pillow-case or hanky is ideal. An unused large plastic bag also works quite well at keeping out the infection, if it is bandaged gently in place. Make sure, however, that it is placed away from the child's face or head. If the child has been burnt in this area, DO NOT use a plastic bag.

● DO NOT break any blisters that may have formed, or peel off any skin. This will only let infection into the burn, making it harder for it to heal without scarring.

● DO NOT put any lotions, potions, ointment or oils on the burn, no matter what, or how tempted you might be to use 'magic cures'. Just cover with the dry dressing and leave until the child reaches hospital.

● DO NOT remove the dressing once you have put it on – not even to see if the skin is blistering and no matter how much you want to re-assure yourself. Just leave the burn alone – fiddling makes it worse.

● DO NOT put any sort of sticking plaster on any but the smallest burn (less than the size of a two-pence piece), because if the skin is burnt, when you peel off the plaster you'll peel off the skin.

Treat for shock

Shock is one of the most dangerous complications that can happen to a child who has been burnt and you need to be on the look-out for it. If there is a sudden loss of fluid of any kind, and this is common in severe burns, the pressure of the blood drops and it can't reach the vital organs (see Chapter 27 on Shock). This is very serious.

REMEMBER – SHOCK LOOKS LIKE THIS

● Her face may be very pale and grey-looking

● Her skin may feel cold and clammy

● Her pulse may feel fast and weak

● She may be frightened and fidgety

● She may be very thirsty

● She may yawn and 'gasp' for air

● She may say everything feels fuzzy

● She may become unconscious

81

If shock occurs, the child will become very quiet, and will look pale and grey. She may say she is feeling sick and she may vomit. When you touch her, her skin will feel cool and clammy. Her pulse will be weak and fast and her breathing will be shallow. She may seem as if she is 'gasping' for air and she may yawn a lot. This is not a sign that she is tired, but that she is starved of oxygen and her condition is serious.

All these signs and symptoms should warn you that the child needs medical help URGENTLY.

● Reassure her. Remember, panic makes things worse. You must stay calm, for her sake.

● Tell her what you are going to do, then lie her down and roll her gently into the Recovery Position with her body to one side, in case she is sick. Try to move her as little as possible. Pick the side you lie her on carefully so that she does not lie on her burns.

● Raise her legs by propping them up gently on cushions. This may be difficult if they are badly burnt but it is vital to get as much blood as possible circulating back to the heart and brain.

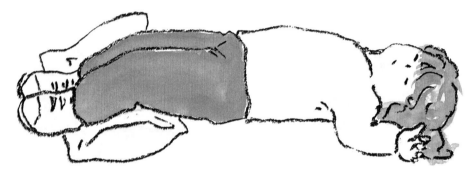

● If she loses consciousness watch her breathing carefully. If it stops, start your ABC Resuscitation Routine.

> **A** for **AIRWAY**   (is it clear?)
>
> **B** for **BREATHING**   (is she breathing?)
>
> **C** for **CIRCULATION**   (is her heart beating?)

● Call for an ambulance by dialling 999. She needs urgent medical help.

In an emergency situation it is always difficult to know when exactly to call the ambulance. Try to attract the attention of a neighbour if you can, and get her to do it for you. Do not leave the child alone, unless it is absolutely necessary. But if you have to, reassure her, and tell her where you are going and what you are going to do. This is not ideal but you may have no choice.

ELECTRICAL BURNS

This happens when the child has an electric shock and the current passes through the body. There is always an 'entry' and 'exit' burn, and although these may appear small and not important, a lot of injury may have been caused underneath the skin or on the path through the body taken by the current.

Electric shocks can be so severe that they cause breathing and/or the child's heart to stop (see Chapter 15 on Electric Shock).

WHAT TO LOOK FOR

There are several things that may make you think a child has had an electric shock:

- She may be lying grasping the socket or appliance or 'exploring object' that she was poking into the appliance.

- She may have been thrown clear of the appliance, for example the toaster, which will be lying nearby.

- There may be a smell of burning flesh, if it is really bad, or of the appliance itself. There may be redness, swelling, scorching or charring of the child's skin.

- The child may be badly shocked (see Chapter 27 on Shock), and could become unconscious.

- The child's heart may have stopped with the strength or frequency of the current. Children are more severely affected than adults by sudden-impact injuries like electric shock. In other words, a shock is more likely to make a child's heart stop than an adult's.

WHAT TO DO

- DO NOT TOUCH THE CHILD until you have removed her from the electricity supply. You can do this either by using dry rubber gloves, a rolled-up newspaper or a wooden stick of some kind to push away the appliance she was touching, or by switching off or disconnecting the electricity supply. If there is no other choice you can kick away the plug or electric appliance she has touched but there is a danger you will be electrocuted unless you are wearing rubber-soled shoes.

- Check that YOU KNOW WHERE THE MAINS SWITCH IS FOR YOUR ELECTRICITY SUPPLY. CAN YOU GET TO IT IN AN EMERGENCY? You may want to think about installing a 'RCD' (Residual Current Device). They can usually 'trip out' a fatal shock before it reaches the child (see Chapter 15 on Electric Shock).

- REMEMBER, if the child loses consciousness you must watch her breathing and if it stops you must start your ABC Resuscitation Routine *before* you do anything else.

> **A** for **AIRWAY**   (is it clear?)
>
> **B** for **BREATHING**   (is she breathing?)
>
> **C** for **CIRCULATION**   (is her heart beating?)

- Constantly reassure the child. There is nothing more terrifying than this sort of injury and she will want to hear your voice and be comforted by it. If she is conscious but too badly hurt to cuddle you, give her a teddy to hold. It might help a little bit.

- Treat her for shock. Remember shock is highly likely in this type of injury. Place her in the Recovery Position, with her body to one side in case she vomits. Try to move her as little as possible. Pick the side you lie her on carefully, being aware of her burns.

- Cool the burn with cold water, but be absolutely sure there is no electricity ANYWHERE around. If there is any doubt skip this stage and go on to the next one.

- DO NOT put anything on the burn except a dry, clean, if possible sterile, non-fluffy dressing or clean plastic bag, held securely but gently in place until the child reaches hospital.

- If you haven't already done so, call the ambulance by dialling 999.

Electrical burns may cause serious internal injury so SHOULD BE SEEN URGENTLY AT HOSPITAL.

CHEMICAL BURNS

These can be caused by everyday things you use in the home, such as oven-cleaners and drain-fluids. These substances may contain strong alkalies (e.g. sodium hydroxide) or strong acids (e.g. hydrochloric acid, found in battery fluid), which if splashed onto a child's skin can be very nasty and cause a serious injury within seconds.

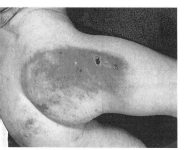

Chemical burn. This is the sort of nasty burn that can be caused by some chemicals.

WHAT TO DO

- Reassure the child. She will be in pain and very frightened. Tell her what you are going to do.

- Hold the limb under cold running water for at least *twenty minutes* or for as long as the child can stand it and gently help her to remove any splashed clothing. If possible put on thick rubber gloves before you take her clothing off, so that you avoid touching the chemical with your bare hands. You can help her more with uninjured hands, so take those few seconds to find some gloves.

- Call an ambulance by dialling 999. Be careful not to leave a small child near a basin or bowl of water in case she faints or falls into the water.

If a child splashes or sprays a chemical liquid or powder in her eye

This is very painful and the child will be distressed. She may be rubbing the eye and it may be swollen or watering a lot.

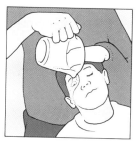

Chemicals in the eye can quickly injure the delicate eye tissue. It is IMPORTANT to stop the burning action. The best way of doing this is by pouring cold water over the eye as soon as possible – but it has to be done in a particular way to stop any more damage being done either to the injured eye or to the other eye.

- If you can, you need to put the child in the 'hairdresser's' position over the sink or basin. It is helpful if someone else can hold her in this position while you gently pour cold running water over from the *inside to the outside* of the eye, either direct from the tap or from a jug. This is easier to do if you encourage the child to look away from the basin. Remember that if you pour from the outside to the inside of the eye, you may wash the chemical back over the other eye.

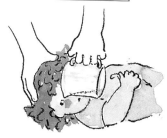

- The best thing to use is an eye-wash bottle (available from specialist chemists – it is also extremely useful for cooling burns and scalds). You fill the bottle with cold water only and this is then sprayed gently into the child's eye to wash out the chemical.

- If the child's eye is closed in spasm, hold it open gently but firmly enough to keep the eye open so that you can splash water in. I'm afraid this is one of those cruel-to-be-kind situations. Most children, too little to understand, will struggle unless first wrapped up firmly in a blanket as their first instinct will be to close the eye and keep it closed. Be careful of long nails when you hold her eye open.

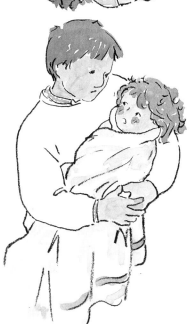

- NEVER use commercial eye-bath solutions. The chemicals may react against those that have splashed in the eye and make the situation worse.

- Don't allow her to rub her eye.

- Cover the injured eye with something clean – sterile if possible.

- Take the child to hospital. Any child with an eye injury should go to hospital where the Accident and Emergency department will give her the emergency treatment she needs (see Chapter 16 on Eye Injuries and Infections).

BURNS TO THE MOUTH AND THROAT

Burns to the mouth and throat are usually caused when a child drinks or eats something that is too hot for her; or swallows a burning-type (corrosive) chemical; or breathes in very hot air, say around a bonfire, when the throat is burnt.

Injuries affecting the throat can be particularly serious in children because the air and food passages are narrower than those in adults. Once burnt, these passages swell up and they can block very quickly. The child then can't swallow or, more important, breathe.

WHAT TO LOOK FOR

There are several things that might make you think she has this kind of injury:

- She may be clutching her throat and gasping.

- She may be finding it difficult to breathe.

- She may be in a state of shock and could become unconscious.

WHAT TO DO

- DO NOT panic. If she sees you panicking, she will too, and that will make her breathe faster, forcing air in and out of an already damaged airway. You must try to comfort and reassure her as much as possible.

- Treat her for shock (see Chapter 27 on Shock).

- Place her in the Recovery Position, with her body on one side, in case she is sick. Try to move her as little possible.

- If she is conscious (for slight *heat* burns only) give her tiny sips of ice-cold water.

- For anything more serious do not give ANYTHING AT ALL TO DRINK. Take her straight to hospital.

Swallowing a corrosive (burning) chemical

- DO NOT make her sick. This will have the effect of burning her twice – once on the way down, and once more on the way up (see Chapter 23 on Poisoning).

- DO NOT give her anything to drink.

- Undo any tight clothing around her neck or take off any necklaces that she is wearing.

- If she becomes unconscious you must watch her breathing and if it stops, start your ABC Resuscitation Routine. If she has swallowed corrosive chemicals, *wipe around her mouth with a cloth before starting mouth-to-mouth respiration* so that you don't burn your mouth too.

A for **AIRWAY** (is it clear?)

B for **BREATHING** (is she breathing?)

C for **CIRCULATION**   (is her heart beating?)

- Get her to hospital as quickly as possible. Dial 999 to get an ambulance, and tell them what has happened.

SUNBURN

If your child has been burnt by the sun, and the skin is swollen and blistered as well as hot, she needs to see a doctor urgently.

Remember that children can burn out of the sun as well as directly underneath it. The danger times are:

- when it is sunny and windy and it is difficult to feel how hot it is;

- when a child has been swimming and her body is wet;

- when a child is floating on the water on an air-bed or with water rings; the water reflects the sun, making it even hotter and therefore more likely to burn her.

WHAT TO DO

Sunburn without hyperthermia

This is when a child has sunburn on the parts of her body that have been exposed to the sun, such as her face, back or legs, and she is *not showing signs of being over-heated* (having hyperthermia).

● Move the child into the shade. Cool her by sponging her skin gently with cool/tepid water. If the child, or, even more important, a baby, has more than one or two blisters or has a large area of sunburn, cool the area by spraying or splashing cold water on to the burns for about fifteen minutes. Then cover with a clean cloth – sterile if possible. Meanwhile call for an ambulance by dialling 999. Tell them what has happened. *she must see a doctor urgently.*

● Reassure and comfort her – she may be in a lot of pain. She may also be in a state of shock (see Chapter 27 on Shock).

> ## REMEMBER – SHOCK LOOKS LIKE THIS
>
> ● Her face may be very pale and grey-looking
>
> ● Her skin may feel cold and clammy
>
> ● Her pulse may feel fast and weak
>
> ● She may be frightened and fidgety
>
> ● She may be very thirsty
>
> ● She may yawn and 'gasp' for air
>
> ● She may say everything feels fuzzy
>
> ● She may become unconscious

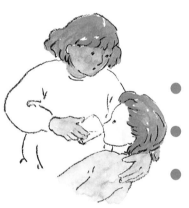

● If she is alert (notices and responds to you) give her lots of *little* sips of water.

● If her breathing is noisy, and she is *not* alert (that is, not aware of your being there) do not give her anything to drink.

● If the child becomes unconscious watch her breathing carefully. If it stops, you must start your ABC Resuscitation Routine immediately.

> **A** for **AIRWAY**   (is it clear?)
>
> **B** for **BREATHING**   (is she breathing?)
>
> **C** for **CIRCULATION**   (is her heart beating?)

Sunburn with hyperthermia

If your child is showing signs of being over-heated (that is she is suffering from hyperthermia) as well as sunburnt, SHE SHOULD BE TAKEN TO HOSPITAL IMMEDIATELY.

This is what a child with hyperthermia will look and feel like:

● In the early stages the child will begin to feel unwell. She will feel dizzy and sick and may vomit.

- She will look flushed and hot (older children may look 'sweaty'). When you put your hand on her tummy it will feel hot and sticky.

- In the later stages of hyperthermia (if, for instance, she has been in the heat for a long time) her skin will be hot and *dry*.

- She may be very restless, her breathing may be noisy and she may become unconscious.

This is an emergency and the child must go to hospital as quickly as possible so that the large amount of fluid that she will have lost from her body can be replaced.

Call for an ambulance, if you haven't already done so, by dialling 999.

General advice

During high summer in the UK, and in a hot climate, never allow a child to sunbathe or stay out in the sun at any time except the early morning and late afternoon. Always cover the skin with sun-protection cream. Factor 12 is a good one for young children, but even so, it needs to be reapplied every few hours and ALWAYS after swimming (even the waterproof kind). If your children are playing outside, please re-member how powerful the sun can be on tender young skins. Always protect young children's heads by making them wear a hat; tie it on if you have to.

If you use sun-ray lamps in your household make sure you spell out the dangers to an older child. NEVER let children use a sun-ray lamp. They are dangerous and, children being children, they are bound to want to experiment when parents are not around. There have been some very bad burning accidents from these lamps. It's very difficult to tell how powerful they are.

MINOR BURNS
- Reassure and talk calmly to the child.
- Cool the burned area in cold water for TEN MINUTES.
- Cover burn with clean dry cloth.
- If burn is bigger than a two-pence piece, see a doctor.

SEVERE BURNS
- If clothing is on fire: STOP – the child from moving around; DROP – the child quickly onto floor; ROLL – the child *onto* the flames and smother with heavy material such as curtains, rug, clothing.
- Protect the child's face.
- Cover the burn with a clean (if possible sterile) cloth.
- Keep splashing cold water onto the cloth. Keep it wet and cold.
- Treat the child for shock. Put her in Recovery Position – turn her away from the burns if possible. Reassure as much as you can.
- Dial 999 for an ambulance. Tell them what has happened.

THINK

- Have you got help? Try shouting at the window or front door.
- Have you checked for DANGER?
- Shake and shout at the child to see if she is conscious.

IF THE CHILD BECOMES UNCONSCIOUS: be ready to start your ABC RESUSCITATION ROUTINE.

Now check 'A' for AIRWAY – is it clear?

IF SHE DOESN'T RESPOND: OPEN THE AIRWAY. Tilt the child's head back and lift her chin foward. REMEMBER babies' necks are chubbier and more fragile. **Be gentle yet firm enough to tilt head back so airway is open.**

Now check 'B' for BREATHING

LOOK
LISTEN } for breathing
FEEL

IF THE CHILD IS NOT BREATHING: BREATHE FOR THE CHILD. Cover her mouth, or nose and mouth, with your mouth. Give her FIVE separate breaths. Watch her chest rise with each breath (*less* breath for babies).

Now check 'C' for CIRCULATION

Is her heart beating? Feel the neck (or arm in a baby) for a pulse.

IF YOU CANNOT FEEL A PULSE: DO CHEST COMPRESSION. Feel for the right place – one finger-breadth below the nipple line. Press on the chest, at a rate of **100 presses per minute**.

For children over one year old: Use the 'heel' of one hand only, with your arm straight. **Press fifteen times to every two breaths** (so your hand presses in about 2.5-3.5cm or 1-1½ inches each time).

For babies: Use two fingers only and **press five times to one breath** (so your fingers press in about 2cm or about ¾ of an inch, each time).

CHOKING

8

Around 20,000 children choke each year and out of these a hundred die. When Esther Rantzen did a *That's Life* item on choking, Dr David Zideman showed what parents should do if their child started to choke. Seven mothers rang up afterwards to say that they had saved their child's life, just by doing exactly what David had demonstrated. I wonder how many parents did not ring up, or how many children have died because their mothers or minders didn't know what to do.

Choking accidents are one of the easiest to treat successfully, and yet so few people know what to do. Choking happens when the airway is blocked or partially blocked by something that may have been meant to go into the tummy or shouldn't have been going near the mouth at all.

There is no doubt that choking is one of the most frightening things that can happen to a child – and to the adult watching her.

The children most at risk from these sorts of accidents tend to be under three years of age. However, *children from four to eleven years are more likely to inhale pen tops*. Please warn your children NOT to put these in their mouth. (They tend to do this when they are absorbed in something they are writing or drawing.) Try also to buy pens with air vents in the top so that if they are accidentally inhaled the child may still be able to breathe enough until the object is removed in hospital.

WHAT TO LOOK FOR

It is easy to recognise a child who is choking. Her face is red at first with the effort to breathe, and the veins on her face stand out. But as the airway becomes more obstructed the skin becomes paler and the lips, tips of ears and nose become a bluish colour. This is because as breathing becomes more difficult the amount of oxygen getting to the lungs and therefore the rest of the body is reduced.

In many accidents it is the sheer terror of the situation that makes it seem so much worse. This applies particularly to choking because the spasm of the muscles at the back of the throat can be caused by the *fear* of not being able to breathe. The more the child fights for breath the more the muscles will go into spasm. You may be able to persuade an older child to cough; this might help to stop the spasm, and stop the choking.

While the child is spluttering she may not be in any immediate danger because the air is still getting in through the airway. However, if you think the airway is becoming blocked you will have to ACT QUICKLY OR SHE MAY STOP BREATHING.

WHAT TO DO

Before you begin any first aid always tell the child, as calmly as you can, exactly what you are going to do so that she doesn't panic. Any panicking automatically makes breathing more difficult and cuts down the amount of oxygen that the child is trying to breathe in.

If you think the child has something stuck in her throat, then, one way or another, you have to turn her so that her *head is lower than her feet*. In other words, you need gravity to help you get it out.

Babies and children under one year

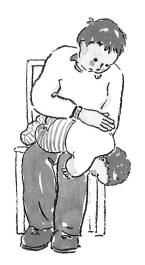

● Hold a baby or very small child head downwards over your forearm, supporting the chest with the arm and the back with your hand. Slap smartly between the shoulder blades *five times*. Almost always the slap will move the object enough for the child to be able to cough it out.

● Check that nothing has come flying out of the mouth onto the floor, and that nothing has come into the mouth from the throat.

● If the stuck object does not come out, you must GET MEDICAL HELP URGENTLY. Take the child with you to the telephone and dial 999.

● If the child becomes unconscious watch her carefully, and if she stops breathing you must start your ABC Resuscitation Routine.

> **A** for **AIRWAY**   (is it clear?)
>
> **B** for **BREATHING**   (is she breathing?)
>
> **C** for **CIRCULATION**   (is her heart beating?)

If the child is unconscious, the muscles around the airway will probably relax enough to allow you to blow air past the blockage, and into the lungs.

Children over one year

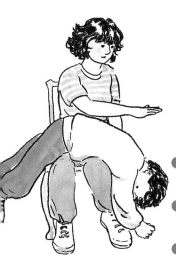

● If the child is small enough to lift, put her head down over your knee. Slap her sharply between the shoulder blades, up to five times.

● Check that nothing has come flying out of the mouth onto the floor, and that nothing has come into the mouth from the throat.

● If the stuck object does not come out, you must GET MEDICAL HELP URGENTLY. Carry or, if you have to, drag the child with you to the telephone and dial 999 for an ambulance.

Meanwhile if you still have not cleared the airway there are two other things you *must* do:

If the child is becomes unconscious watch her carefully, and if she stops breathing you must start your ABC Resuscitation Routine.

A for **AIRWAY**   (is it clear?)

B for **BREATHING**   (is she breathing?)

C for **CIRCULATION**   (is her heart beating?)

If the child is unconscious, the muscles around the airway will relax enough to allow you to blow air past the blockage, and into the lungs.

If the airway stays blocked, you must try the 'abdominal thrust'. *This is a tricky thing to do but without it your child might die.* There is a danger that, however careful you are, you might do some damage to the organs inside her abdomen – but we are talking about life and death and at this stage you don't really have a choice.

You are going to squeeze the tummy sharply and quickly to make her cough. Sit the child on your lap with her head as low as possible so that gravity will help to get the object out. Place your arm around her middle and make a fist with your thumb tucked in. Place your fist in the middle of the top part of the tummy. Put the other hand over the first hand and press the clenched fist into the tummy. Pull sharply inwards and upwards towards the child's back.

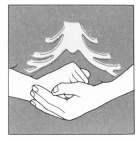

Close-up of hand position for abdominal thrust in a *conscious* child.

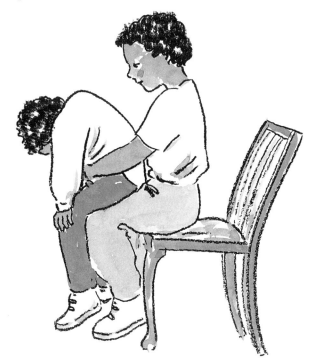

The thrust must be strong enough to force out the object that is stuck in the windpipe. After each thrust, check to see that nothing has come flying out of the mouth on to the floor, and that nothing has come into the mouth from the throat.

If it doesn't work, then try it again – up to five times. Then try five back-slaps (described above). If the object still hasn't moved try five thrusts and so on until the ambulance arrives. BE AWARE that this manoeuvre could injure a child, particularly if she is very little, as it might cause internal injury. But you may have to use it to save your child's life. DON'T TRY THIS TECHNIQUE ON BABIES – IT IS TOO DANGEROUS.

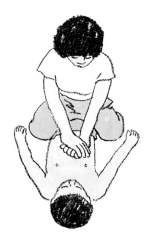

● IF THE CHILD IS UNCONSCIOUS (or becomes unconscious while you are trying to get the object out of her windpipe), you must quickly try the 'abdominal thrust' in a different way.

Roll the child onto her side and give five back-slaps. If this doesn't work, then turn her onto her back with her head tilted back to open the airway.

Kneel astride her so that you have enough control to put firm pressure on the middle of her tummy when you lean forward. Place the heel of one hand in the centre of the top part of the child's tummy and *lift your fingers up* to lessen any chance of internal injury, then put your other hand over the first.

Hold the arms straight, thrust sharply and firmly *upwards* towards the diaphragm. This must be hard enough to make the child cough out the object that is stuck in the windpipe.

If the object is still stuck, don't give up. Try again – up to another five times. Then try five back-slaps (described above). Check that nothing has come flying out of the mouth onto the floor, or that nothing has come into the mouth from the throat. Check her breathing. If the object still hasn't moved try five thrusts and so on until the ambulance arrives.

Carry on with your ABC Resuscitation Routine until the ambulance arrives so that you continue to get oxygen into and around her body. You can only do that by breathing for her and by trying chest compression with your hands on her chest so that the blood circulates to the most important places – the heart, lungs and brain.

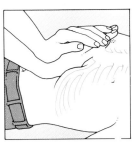

Close-up of hand position for abdominal thrust in an *unconscious* child.

- Talk *calmly* to the child.
- Hold the baby or child *over your knee* – head down.
- Slap sharply up to five times, between the shoulder blades, using the flat of your hand.
- After each slap, *check that nothing has come out of the mouth.*
- Dial 999 (you may have to take the child with you to the phone).

THINK

- Have you got help? Try shouting at window or front door.
- Have you called the ambulance? Try to get someone to do this for you.
- Shake and shout to the child to see if she is conscious.

IF THE CHILD BECOMES UNCONSCIOUS: be ready to start your ABC RESUSCITATION ROUTINE.

Now check   'A' for AIRWAY – is it clear?

IF SHE DOESN'T RESPOND: OPEN THE AIRWAY. Tilt the child's head back and lift her chin forward. REMEMBER babies' necks are chubbier and more fragile. **Be gentle yet firm enough to tilt head back so airway is open.**

Now check   'B' for BREATHING

LOOK
LISTEN } for breathing
FEEL

IF THE CHILD IS NOT BREATHING: BREATHE FOR THE CHILD. Cover her mouth, or nose and mouth, with your mouth. Give her FIVE separate breaths. Watch her chest rise with each breath. *Less* breath for babies.

Now check   'C' for CIRCULATION

Is her heart beating? Feel the neck (or arm in a baby) for a pulse.

IF YOU CANNOT FEEL A PULSE: DO CHEST COMPRESSION. Feel for the right place – one finger-breadth below the nipple line. Press on the chest, at a rate of **100 presses per minute.**

For children over one year old: Use the 'heel' of one hand only, with your arm straight. **Press fifteen times to every two breaths** (so your hand presses in about 2.5-3.5cm or 1-1½ inches each time).

For babies: Use two fingers only and **press five times to one breath** (so your fingers press in about 2cm or about ¾ of an inch, each time).

IF YOU CANNOT BLOW PAST THE OBSTRUCTION – TRY THE ABDOMINAL THRUST (YOU MUST NOT TRY THIS ON BABIES). If *conscious*: sit child on lap, head low. Place your arm around top of her tummy. Make a fist. Put other hand over fist, pull sharply inwards and upwards to force object out. If *unconscious*: roll child onto back. Kneel astride her. Place heel of one hand over top-centre of tummy – lift fingers up. Put other hand on top, hold arms straight. Thrust sharply and firmly upwards towards diaphragm. If this doesn't work, try five back slaps followed by five abdominal thrusts.

KEEP DOING THIS UNTIL THE AMBULANCE ARRIVES.

9 COT DEATH

This chapter is dedicated to the memory of Joshua.

Although cot death is the commonest cause of death in babies up to one year old, it is *still very rare* – only two out of every 1000 children are affected. This doesn't mean that it isn't the most tragic thing that can happen to any parent – but please don't let the worry that it could happen spoil those precious early months with your baby.

The reasons why babies die from cot (infant) death are complicated. Doctors are still not sure why this happens, although all sorts of reasons have been put forward.

The Foundation for the Study of Infant Deaths has written these guidelines which are thought to reduce the risks of cot death:

- Lie your baby on his back or side NOT on his tummy. Some babies, however, are naturally tummy sleepers and keep wriggling back again. But if you keep turning them over and tucking them in securely with their blankets – as long as the weather is not too hot – they will eventually get used to it. (One way to encourage them to do this is to have a mobile hanging over the cot – even a musical one – so that they can gaze at it as they hopefully drift off.)

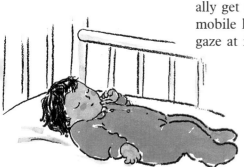

- Your baby should NEVER have a pillow for sleeping (see Chapter 28 on Suffocation). If, however, you want to raise the baby's head because he is a little snuffly and his nose is blocked, you can put a small pillow *under* the cot mattress – but if you raise the head end too much the baby will just slide to the bottom of the cot (see 'Coughs and Colds' in Chapter 22 on Minor Injuries and Illnesses).

- Try not to smoke when you are pregnant. Mothers who smoke tend to have smaller or premature babies and these babies are more at risk from cot death. After the baby has been born, keep him out of smoky rooms. If you smoke, try to do so in a room where the baby doesn't sleep and ask relatives and friends to do the same. It is obviously better for you, and the baby, if you give up smoking.

- Don't let your baby get too hot – or too cold. This is difficult to get right. There is no doubt that in the first month of life babies can catch cold easily and have to be kept warm. Just be careful, if you have the heating on in the house or flat, that you always take his outdoor clothes off once you get inside, especially if it's winter. Once a baby is over a year old he is slightly better at keeping himself warm, but he can't get himself cool again once he gets too hot! At this stage he can wear the same amount of clothes as an adult, as long as you keep him away from draughts, but he has to be *well wrapped up to go outside*, especially in winter. It is still important to take the extra layers off once he comes back inside. No baby should ever wear a hat indoors, it makes them too hot. (Babies gain and lose heat very quickly through their heads.)

● Try to keep the house or flat at an even temperature. This is difficult if you don't have central heating. Don't worry about him getting cold at night – you don't need the heating on then, particularly if the room has been warm during the day. As long as he is wearing nappy, vest and baby-gro (or something similar) and is tucked securely into his blankets, he will be fine. It is important that he doesn't get too hot at night.

● DO NOT use a sheepskin (no matter how tempting the manufacturers make it sound – see Chapter 28 on Suffocation) or a hot-water bottle for any baby. Both are dangerous.

● It is difficult to know how many blankets to put on the cot, but it will depend on what sort of blankets you use and how warm or cold the room is at night. See the chart on page 184, which is a guide to how many blankets you might use.

● Duvets, baby nests and cot bumpers are not recommended for babies under one year old. The baby may suffocate (see Chapter 28 on Suffocation).

If you want to be really sure that the baby is warm enough, you may want a bedroom and nursery thermometer. These can be purchased from:

The Foundation for the Study of Infant Deaths
35 Belgrave Square, London SW1X 8QB.
The price at time of writing is £2.50.

The other way to tell whether your baby is warm enough is to feel his tummy – make sure your hands are warm before you do it though! Hands and feet may be cold but if his tummy is warm he really is all right.

When your baby seems to be ill, you need to watch him very carefully. Some babies seem to get a few coughs and snuffles, with or without a small rise in temperature, and cope with them very well. Others can get very ill very quickly. Unfortunately you don't know how your baby will react so you have to be on your guard every time.

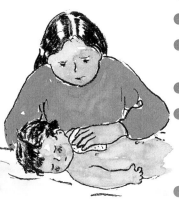

If your baby has a temperature of 39°C (102°F) or over (see 'Fever' in Chapter 22 on Minor Injuries and Illnesses):

- You must cool him down, but not too quickly.

- Turn the heating down or take him away from a sunny window.

- Remove the blankets and covers from his cot and, if his temperature is high, his baby-gro as well.

- Sponge him down with tepid (not cold, not hot) water.

- Give him lots to drink. It is even a good idea to wake him up to give him a drink. Ill babies often sleep a lot and if they sleep too long, and they have a temperature, they can get dehydrated – in other words, they lose too much fluid from their bodies.

- He may need medicine such as paracetamol-syrup to help to bring his temperature down. The correct dose for a baby is written clearly on the bottle. All medicine is different, so check the dose before you give it. NEVER give an adult preparation. Try to use one which is sugar-free.

- If the baby is very young, or if you are worried, call the doctor.

Always ask for help and advice from your midwife, Health Visitor or doctor. That is what they are there for and they would much rather be called unnecessarily than not called when it might be serious. You may be too tired or too busy to know for sure if your baby is ill, especially if you have got other children needing your attention.

Most Health Visitors, for instance, don't mind being 'bothered' if you ring them up because you are worried. Between 9 a.m. and 10 a.m. or 4 p.m. and 5 p.m. is best, otherwise they are usually out on calls. They will certainly come in for a cup of coffee and a chat.

You must be able to recognise the signs which are serious. If your baby appears to stop breathing or goes blue, you need to know if he is conscious. One way to find this out is to *shake your baby gently* and *shout at him*. If he is conscious he will respond – if only to cry.

If he doesn't respond, YOU NEED TO GET EXPERT HELP URGENTLY. Don't try to cope by yourself. If you can, get someone to call for an ambulance by dialling 999. Make sure that whoever calls for it knows the number of your house or flat. Tell them the baby has stopped breathing.

If you are on your own in the house carry the baby with you to the telephone. If there is no phone in the house, go to the front doorstep and shout for help.

While the ambulance is on its way to you, they may take you through the things that you must do to save your baby's life. Try to listen carefully to what they are telling you.

Meanwhile start your ABC Resuscitation Routine.

> **A** for **AIRWAY**   (is it clear?)
>
> **B** for **BREATHING**   (is he breathing?)
>
> **C** for **CIRCULATION**   (is his heart beating?)

A for Airway

You need to know if the airway is clear.

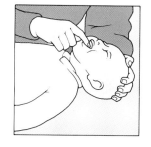

- Carry the baby to a table or some other firm surface. If it has to be the floor you won't have as much control as you would at table level. With one hand on the forehead, and the first finger of the other hand on the bony part of the chin, tilt the head back, grip the chin and lift it forward.

  In a baby the neck is shorter and chubbier than in older children. You need to be careful not to push the head too far back. On the other hand it is vital that the short airway is opened up as far as it will go.

- Look inside the mouth to see if there is anything obvious blocking the airway. If it's the tongue, for instance, when you pull up the chin to free the airway, there may be a choking sound and you will know immediately that he has started breathing again.

  If you think you can see a lump of vomit, food or small object, then try to scoop it out with your little finger.

  DON'T stick your finger blindly down his throat, you could do more damage by pushing any object further down.

- Check the nostrils. Babies and small children tend to breathe through their nostrils, and if they are blocked this can make a difficult situation worse. If, however, you feel there is nothing obvious blocking his airway, move quickly to B.

B for Breathing

- *If breathing stops there is no oxygen getting to the brain.* Within THREE MINUTES the brain cells begin to die. It is vital that you take urgent action to restart the baby's breathing as soon as you possibly can.

  The three things to remember are:

1 **LOOK**

2 **LISTEN** } for breathing

3 **FEEL**

Do all of these by placing your ear over the baby's mouth to:

LOOK along the outline of his chest, to see if his chest is rising and falling, as it normally does when we breathe.

LISTEN for breathing sounds.

FEEL for breath coming out of his mouth or nostrils onto the side of your face. Spend about five seconds doing this. His breath may be very shallow and you may not be able to feel it at first. If breathing has stopped, then you must act quickly and breathe for the baby in order to fill the air sacs of the lungs with air. This is called Artificial Respiration (see Chapter 3 on ABC Resuscitation Routine). If you are not sure whether or not his breathing has stopped take a chance and start to breathe for him anyway.

● When you are breathing for a baby remember three things:

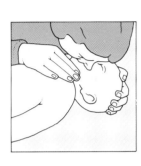

1 Cover the baby's *mouth and nose* to get a better flow of air into the airway.

2 The neck is shorter, chubbier and more fragile than in older children. Be gentle, yet firm enough to tilt the head back so that the airway is open, otherwise no air can get through.

3 Blow until you see the chest start to rise.

● Remember: DON'T BLOW TOO HARD. There is a danger that air could be blown into the tummy, causing the food inside to spill over into the lungs.

● GIVE FIVE SEPARATE BREATHS, enough to make his chest rise each time. Take your mouth away after each breath. As you breathe into the baby, LOOK along the outside of his chest, to see if it is rising with each breath. If it is, this means that the air you are breathing in is travelling down the airway and into the tiny air sacs in the lungs. It is only by reaching these air sacs that the exchange of gases (oxygen and carbon dioxide) can take place.

If the chest does not rise the most likely reason is that the airway is not fully open, so look again at the position of his head and see if you can *gently* lift the chin up or tilt the head back a bit more. It is only by adjusting the airway and straightening out any kinks that you can get the correct position and allow air to pass through more easily.

If this doesn't work then the baby may have something stuck in the airway (see Chapter 8 on Choking).

C for Circulation

The whole purpose of resuscitation is to KEEP THE BRAIN ALIVE.

Once the heart slows or stops, it takes only *three minutes* before the brain cells begin to die and brain damage takes place. Whether you do this or the heart does, doesn't matter. What matters is getting the blood circulating again urgently and as efficiently as possible.

● After giving the first five breaths into the baby's mouth and nose, you must immediately check to see if the heart is working. There is no point in breathing for him *if the air is not being circulated around the body.*

- The way to find out is to feel for the pulse. The carotid (neck) pulse is the strongest in the body but it may be difficult to find in an infant because the neck is short and chubby. An easier one, therefore, is the brachial pulse, found on the inside of the upper arm, midway between the elbow and the shoulder. Press your two forefingers gently towards the bone, while holding the outside of the arm with your thumb.

  It is a good idea to 'practise' on your own baby, so that you know where the pulse is and what it feels like. It is often difficult to do for the first time in an emergency. (You may feel it is tempting fate – I just think it is sensible.) You can also feel the brachial pulse in adults (not as strongly as in the neck) and it might be easier to practise this way.

  If you think you cannot feel a pulse don't take any chances, begin chest compression immediately. This means pressing the chest so that the blood – with its vital oxygen – is pumped around the body and up to the brain.

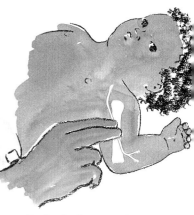

Feeling for the arm pulse in a baby (brachial).

- Place two fingers just below the nipple line in the middle of his chest and press down firmly, so that your fingers press in about ½ to 1 inch (1.25 to 2.5cm). REMEMBER what you are trying to do is to press his chest *just hard enough* to pump blood (and therefore oxygen) around his body and up to his brain. Hopefully the heart (which is the size of the baby's tiny closed fist) will then start to beat again by itself.

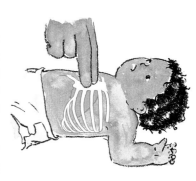

- PRESS FIRMLY FIVE TIMES at the rate of 100 beats per minute or three times every two seconds (that is, slightly quicker than one press every second). Then *give the baby one breath*, using mouth-to-mouth-nose breathing (see B for Breathing above). Then repeat the whole sequence: press his chest five times, then give him one breath. Continue this Resuscitation Routine until help arrives.

REMEMBER, WHETHER IT IS A BABY OR A CHILD WHO STOPS BREATHING, THE SOONER YOU CAN BEGIN RESUSCITATION THE BETTER CHANCE YOU HAVE OF SAVING HIS LIFE.

- *You need to get expert medical help urgently.* If you haven't done so already, call for an ambulance by dialling 999. Continue breathing for your baby and giving him chest compressions. Tell the emergency operator what you are trying to do.

- While the ambulance is on its way to you, they may take you through the resuscitation technique so that you don't feel that you are coping on your own with a baby who isn't breathing.

- KEEP RESUSCITATING UNTIL THE AMBULANCE ARRIVES.

The *Safe and Sound* video of this technique may help you to understand it even better (see page 284 for details).

If you think your baby is ill, never hesitate to call the doctor.

Doctors would rather see a baby whose parent or carer thinks is ill, and isn't, than a very ill baby whose parent didn't realise and may have left it too late.

The Foundation for the Study of Infant Deaths (FSID) is a special organisation set up to research the causes of cot death. You may have had a cot death in your family and are worried about the next baby; or perhaps you know someone whose baby died in this way. Whatever the reason, they will try to help you. You will get comfort, reassurance and the latest information from them. They also produce a very helpful leaflet called *Reduce the Risk of Cot Death*. Write to:

The Foundation for the Study of Infant Deaths
35 Belgrave Square, London SW1X 8QB.
Tel. 071 235 0965

Or you can phone:

The Cot Death Helpline 071 235 1721

IF YOU THINK YOUR BABY HAS STOPPED BREATHING, YOU NEED URGENT MEDICAL HELP:

THINK

- Can you get some help? Try shouting out of the window or front door.
- Have you called the ambulance? Try to get someone to do this for you.
- Shake and shout to the child to see if he is conscious.

Start your ABC RESUSCITATION ROUTINE.

Now check   'A' for AIRWAY – is it clear?

IF HE DOESN'T RESPOND: OPEN THE AIRWAY. REMEMBER babies' necks are chubby and fragile. **Be gentle yet firm enough to tilt head back so airway is open.**

Now check   'B' for BREATHING

LOOK
LISTEN } for breathing
FEEL

IF THE BABY IS NOT BREATHING: BREATHE FOR THE BABY. Cover his nose and mouth, with your mouth. Give him FIVE separate breaths – they may be no more than light puffs – but **enough to make his chest rise with each breath.**

Now check   'C' for CIRCULATION

Is his heart beating? Check for the pulse. Feel the arm for his pulse. **If there is no pulse and you haven't got help GET IT NOW.**

IF YOU CANNOT FEEL A PULSE: DO CHEST COMPRESSION. Feel for the right place – one finger-breadth below the nipple line. Press on the chest, at a rate of **100 presses per minute. Use two fingers only and press five times to one breath** (so your fingers press in about 2cm which is about ¾ of an inch, each time).

KEEP DOING THIS UNTIL THE AMBULANCE ARRIVES.

10 CROUP

Seeing and hearing a child having an attack of croup can be one of the most alarming experiences for parents or anyone who is looking after the child. Attacks usually occur at night, often suddenly, and the child will wake up with a distinctive, hollow, barking cough. It is difficult to describe, but once you have heard it, you will recognise it as croup.

The child may have difficulty getting her breath. She may have 'lost her voice' and been unable to call you, and she will be scared by the peculiar noise she is making in her throat. She will probably have a temperature, possibly a high one.

Croup is the childhood version of laryngitis. Adults tend to get a tickly throat and just put up with it; but children's air passages are narrower and when they get an infection, perhaps a cold or sore throat, it goes into the voice box and down the windpipe. The delicate lining of these air passages then swells up and the danger is that they will block up completely. It is the sound of the air being sucked in or forced out through the swollen voice box, as the child breathes, that makes the 'croupy' sound. (See page 25 on How the Body Works.)

This is an emergency and you have to ACT QUICKLY.

DO NOT in any circumstances stick anything into the child's mouth to 'have a look' down her throat. Very rarely, instead of the voice box, the epiglottis becomes inflamed and swells up. This is the lid covering the voice box during swallowing – it stops food and drink 'going down the wrong way'. This is a very dangerous condition. If you stick anything in the child's mouth – the end of a spoon for instance – as you might if she says she has a sore throat, *you could block her airway completely*.

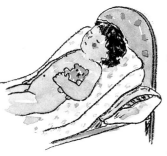

WHAT TO DO

● Calm and reassure the child. She is short of oxygen, because of her difficulty in breathing. The more she panics and struggles the more oxygen she needs. Take a few seconds to cuddle her and then tell her what you are going to do. This will comfort the child and allow you to think about what you *are* going to do.

● Try and get her to sit up and lean forward, if she is big enough to understand, otherwise just prop her up on pillows. If she is very little put them *underneath* the head end of the mattress to raise it.

● If the child has a temperature, you need to get it down (see 'Fever' in Chapter 22 on Minor Injuries and Illnesses on taking a temperature). It may be difficult at this stage to get any medicine into her, but if you can, a paracetamol-syrup will help to bring the temperature down quickly. If she won't take it, and you feel that by trying to give it to her it will only make things worse, then just take off her night-clothes for the time being. Don't forget to tell her why you are doing this, otherwise it may upset her even more.

Steam up a small room because warm damp air is a lot easier to breathe than cold dry air. You can do this by turning on all the hot taps in the bathroom – making sure the door and window are firmly closed – or by boiling an electric kettle and keeping your finger on the 'on' button (it is much better if you do this in a small room).

If you are using a kettle *make sure it is full when you boil it* and keep checking that there is enough water in it, and that the water level does not fall below the level of the element (the pipes at the bottom of the kettle), otherwise it may burn.

REMEMBER *this steam is hot and very dangerous to a child* (or to you) if the hot steam is breathed in.

If you have anyone with you in the house, ask them to prepare a room full of steam.

Take her to the steamy room. If you haven't got anyone with you in the house, take the child with you as you prepare the room or get the kettle.

Stay there for as long as it takes her to breathe more easily. You will know this because the croupy noise will get less and she will appear calmer. She will generally seem to be a lot happier and may take a drink, and her colour will look better. But be prepared to go back if it starts again.

Please BE AWARE that the croupy sound easing off may also be a danger sign as it could mean the child is breathing in less air.

Try to reduce her temperature further by sponging her with tepid (not warm, not cold) water, particularly under the arms and behind her neck. See if you can now get her to take a paracetamol-syrup – this will help to get her temperature down quickly and generally make her feel better (see 'Fever' in Chapter 22 on Minor Injuries and Illnesses).

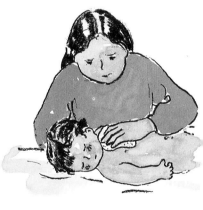

Call for the doctor (if you haven't already) and explain what has happened, taking the child with you to the telephone if you are alone.

Do not leave your child alone for a moment in a steamy room. The source of the steam will be boiling hot and dangerous to a child – whether it is the electric kettle or the hot taps. *Even when the doctor arrives take the child with you* to open the door.

If the doctor can't come immediately or if the child seems to be getting worse, dial 999 for an ambulance. Tell them what has happened.

Alternatively you may want to take her to your nearest Accident and

105

Emergency department. If you are on your own with her in the house, see if you can ask a neighbour or friend to drive you to the hospital while you hold her. Don't try to drive yourself. If there is no one to help, wait for the ambulance.

You can tell if your child is getting worse in the following ways:

- *Her breathing becomes more difficult* – in other words it is becoming more difficult for the air to get through the swollen air passages into the lungs. Her croupy breathing may become quieter.

- *Sucking in of her ribcage.* If her lower chest is being sucked in as she takes a breath, it is a sign that she is having serious difficulty breathing. You must keep checking that this is not happening.

- *Her colour changes.* As the child becomes more distressed the oxygen that is getting to her lungs is reduced. Her usually pink lips take on a bluish-grey tone and her skin becomes pale and grey-looking.

- *She will be listless*, taking no interest in anything around her. She will probably refuse drinks and appear not to notice even that you are there.

- If the child becomes unconscious open her airway and check her breathing. If it stops, you must start your ABC Resuscitation Routine.

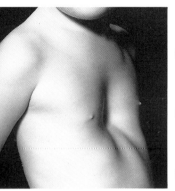

Sucking in of the ribcage. This is what a child looks like when her breathing is severely affected by croup. This child needs urgent admission to hospital.

> **A** for **AIRWAY**   (is it clear?)
>
> **B** for **BREATHING**   (is she breathing?)
>
> **C** for **CIRCULATION**   (is her heart beating?)

The difficulty of resuscitating a child with swollen air passages is that you might not be able to get any air through into the lungs. *Try therefore to watch out for any of the danger signs and get this child to hospital as quickly as you can.*

If your child gets croup again

One of the most distressing things about children who have had croup is that they seem to get it again whenever they have a sore throat, and unfortunately every time is an emergency.

You have to be prepared, so that if an attack starts in the middle of the night (and you rarely get any warning), you know what to do.

- Invest in a steam vaporiser. You can buy an electric one, which is expensive but worthwhile if you have a child who gets frequent attacks. Or you can buy a cheaper coal-tar vaporiser which also works very well. It heats the vaporiser fluid which is poured into an absorbent block at the top.

- Keep a bottle of paracetamol-syrup in your medicine cupboard (that is in a place out of the reach of children), and know the dose to give, in case she has a high temperature.

- Be ready to make a steamy room. Decide beforehand how you are going to do this. Then once her breathing has eased you can put her in her bedroom with the vaporiser on. (Get it ready, or switch it on, as soon as the attack starts, then as soon as she has been in the intense steam, she can go back to bed.)

- While she is in the steamy room try to bring her temperature down by sponging her with tepid water (see above).

- Sit her up in bed with plenty of pillows. If she is very little put the pillows *under* the head end of the mattress.

- It might be useful to make a few notes about what happened and helped the previous time. It will save the hassle of thinking out what to do on each occasion.

- Have a mattress and sleeping bag or bedclothes near at hand so that you can move into her room if you have to. It is not a good idea to leave a croupy child alone, particularly if your room is not within earshot of hers. You need to keep an eye – and an ear – on her, even if the attack is a mild one.

- Never be afraid of phoning the doctor, no matter what time of night it is or how many times you have called him before for a croup attack.

EACH TIME is an emergency and your doctor will understand.

Vaporisers, either manual or electric, can be purchased from most big chemists. The prices range (at the time of writing) from about £10 for the candle-lit one (manual) to between £20 and £95 for an electric one. The £95 one gives you steam control – you can have as much or as little as you need. All the electric ones have the choice of hot or cold steam.

If you are unable to find a vaporiser in chemists near you, you can buy them from:

John Bell and Croyden
50 Wigmore Street, London W1.
Tel. 071 935 5555
If you cannot call at the shop they can send it to you by mail order.

- Calm and reassure the child.
- Sit her up on pillows and lean her forward.
- 'Steam up' a small room. DO NOT *leave the child in there alone*.
- Ring for the doctor and say it is urgent.

IF THE CHILD'S CONDITION GETS WORSE, THIS IS WHAT TO LOOK FOR:
- Her breathing will be more difficult – it may become quieter.
- There will be 'sucking' in of her ribcage.
- Her skin will change to a blue/greyish colour.
- The child will be listless – show no interest in anything around her and may not notice that you are there.

IF your child has any of these symptoms, ring for an ambulance immediately by dialling 999. DON'T WAIT. Tell them what has happened and that it is an emergency.

THINK

- Have you managed to get some help? Try shouting out of the window or front door.
- Have you called the ambulance? Try to get someone to do this for you.

DO NOT UNDER ANY CIRCUMSTANCES PUT ANYTHING IN YOUR CHILD'S MOUTH IN AN ATTEMPT TO LOOK DOWN HER THROAT.

THIS IS AN EMERGENCY. YOU MUST GET THIS CHILD TO HOSPITAL AS QUICKLY AS YOU CAN.

DIABETES

Diabetic children look and act like other childen and they ARE like other children – except that they may have a slightly dodgy pancreas (see Chapter 2 on How the Body Works).

There are now more children under five years old being diagnosed as having diabetes than ever before.

Diabetes mellitus is due to lack of insulin, a hormone which controls the amount of sugar (glucose) in the blood. The pancreas, which normally keeps the balance between sugar and insulin, doesn't cope very well with the level of sugar in the diabetic child's blood. As the level rises, it makes the child ill. If the child does not receive treatment she will become unconscious and without treatment could even die. The first signs are thirst and passing a lot of urine and she will develop an acetone/pear drop smell on her breath.

A diabetic child, therefore, has to have injections of insulin – under her skin (subcutaneously) – at least once a day. This keeps her blood-sugar level fairly normal. As well as this she has to control her diet and balance the sort of food she eats with the activity she takes.

Children usually have injections, and NOT tablets, to stabilise their diabetes, and have to watch what they eat. Their bodies are growing and they are altogether too unstable to take insulin in any other way than by injection.

Generally, once the child has been stabilised – when the doctors have worked out *exactly* how much food and insulin *this particular child* needs to balance her blood-sugar levels – she should be all right. The dangers come when meals are not taken on time, the child eats too much or too little of the things that she is supposed to, when she takes more exercise than she usually does, or when she has an infection or illness of some sort.

However, if childhood diabetes is handled sensibly and calmly by parents, teachers and other carers – with *lots of communication and sharing of information* – there is no reason why the child shouldn't lead a normal life.

About one child in 900 has diabetes but most teachers and other carers don't come into contact with it often enough to feel really confident in dealing with it if things go wrong.

If your child is told she has diabetes you MUST share any information you have with teachers and other people who look after her – even if it is only for short periods during the week for groups such as Brownies and Cubs. There, children are often dashing around using more energy (and therefore more glucose) in a shorter amount of time than they normally would. Pack leaders ought to know what to do if the child becomes unwell.

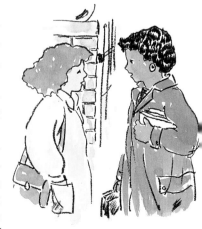

PLEASE DON'T ASSUME THEY KNOW WHAT TO DO. It is possible they may never have met a diabetic child before and they need as much information as they can get.

However, it is not just insulin, diet or exercise that can make the child's blood-sugar levels go out of sync. The onset of an illness like flu, a tummy bug, or even a cold, can change the balance dramatically, as can worry caused by a change of school, exams or any excitement before birthdays or holidays. As for boy/girlfriends – when the time comes – that is when you have to be on your guard. All those hormones whizzing around are enough to upset the most stable children – not eating, putting on/taking off weight, disco dancing till all hours, and so on – and if you have diabetes it can make life a bit tricky. So she and you have to be aware of any problems that might arise – and what to do about them if they do.

If the body does go out of balance, with either too much or too little sugar, the child will become either *hyper*glycaemic (high sugar) or *hypo*-glycaemic (low sugar). Both these problems are fairly easy to recognise and both need urgent attention.

HYPOGLYCAEMIA

This is when there is too little sugar in the blood. If the child becomes 'hypo' it happens alarmingly quickly – particularly if a meal or a snack is delayed, or if she has done a lot of exercise and not taken a snack beforehand.

WHAT TO LOOK FOR

This is what she will look and feel like:

- Some children have their own particular 'thing' which makes them realise that they are becoming 'hypo'. Some have a special kind of headache, or a peculiar sick feeling.

- She will become pale, and seem faint or dizzy.

- Her skin will feel *cold* and she will be *sweating* a lot.

- She may tremble, become confused or even aggressive, or just not be 'herself'.

- She may find it difficult to answer simple questions, or follow simple commands.

- Her breathing will be shallow, in other words almost panting, but her breath will NOT have a smell. If her blood-sugar level is too high, her breath has a very definite smell (see below, Hyperglycaemia).

● If at this stage she is not looked after and given what she needs quickly, which is some sugary snack or drink, *she may become unconscious.*

● *Very* occasionally the child will have a fit (see Chapter 17 on Fits).

The child usually recognises the first clues that she is becoming 'hypo', unless of course she is a new diabetic. (It takes quite a long time to get used to having it.) DO NOT ignore a child who tells you that she is feeling this way, OR if you see her looking a bit peculiar, OR if you see a child who you know has diabetes who looks or feels hypo – *if she looks as though she might be becoming hypo you must assume that she is.* Never take a chance of seeing how she is later, even if you think she *might* be playing up – it's just not worth it.

If she has been diagnosed as diabetic she will have been guided by the doctor about what snack she should take. Some children have a banana, others a mini chocolate bar or a drink of milk, particularly before exercise.

The child should carry a packet of glucose sweets or sugar lumps everywhere she goes. Teachers and part-time carers of a diabetic child (like pack leaders and swimming teachers) should have these available too. It is important to make sure these children *always* have an emergency supply – and know WHY and WHERE they carry them. It is one way of making sure your child is safe in someone else's care.

WHAT TO DO

● If the child is still conscious, and can still swallow, immediately give her the glucose tablets, sugar lumps, a sugary drink (a glucose drink is ideal but remember, low-calorie drinks are no use) or some other sweet food. If she feels, or seems, a bit better give her some more.

● The child must then see the doctor, to see why her insulin injection was too high to cope with the sugar in her body at that time. He will want to test her blood and urine for blood sugar.

● *If she becomes unconscious,* make sure her airway is clear and she is breathing normally. Put her in the Recovery Position but be prepared to do your ABC Resuscitation Routine if breathing stops.

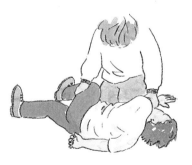

> **A** for **AIRWAY** (is it clear?)
>
> **B** for **BREATHING** (is she breathing?)
>
> **C** for **CIRCULATION** (is her heart beating?)

● Call for an ambulance by dialling 999. Tell them it is urgent and that the child *is in a diabetic coma* and is probably hypoglycaemic.

When a diabetic child becomes unwell at school, *she should never be sent to the medical room on her own.* Please explain this to the teacher. Also make sure you leave your telephone number (or your partner/friend/neighbour's telephone number) where someone can be contacted in an emergency. If the child needs to be sent home the school must be sure that a responsible person will be there to look after her.

A CHILD THOUGHT TO BE HYPO WILL BE HYPO AND SHOULD NEVER BE SENT HOME ALONE.

HYPERGLYCAEMIA

This is when there is too much sugar in the blood. If the child becomes 'hyper' *it happens slowly,* so generally speaking parents and carers have time to realise what is happening – but the child might not, and this of course is the danger. It is much more common for a diabetic child to become hypo- than hyperglycaemic (once she has been diagnosed as having diabetes). These are often the first signs that your child might have diabetes.

WHAT TO LOOK FOR

This is what the child will look and feel like:

● The child will begin to feel more and more 'unwell'.

● She will be very thirsty, no matter how much she drinks.

● She will want to go to the toilet a lot – much more than she does normally.

● She will feel sleepy and drowsy, she may fall asleep in lessons, or not want to get up in the morning.

● She may be sick.

● Her skin will feel hot and dry, and she will look flushed.

● Her breath will smell of pear drops or acetone (nail varnish remover). It is a 'hot, sticky-sweet' breath and once you have smelled it you will recognise it again. Doctors call it a 'ketotic' breath, because what you can smell are the ketones (the 'poisons', that mostly diabetics have), which are being breathed out of her body.

If all of this goes unnoticed she will eventually become unconscious.

WHAT TO DO

- If she hasn't ever seen a doctor about these symptoms, she really should be seen by her GP.

- Ask the child if she has been taking her insulin injection.

- Ask her if by any chance she has been taking any extra tit-bits of food that she shouldn't have. Maybe it was someone's birthday at school. Maybe she just loves chocolate (other children do, so why shouldn't diabetics?) and the temptation may have been too much. She may have been making a habit of it – children will never understand the dangers of an illness (or an action) as adults do.

  If this happens, try not to be too cross, no matter how panicky you might feel. Just try to explain the importance of it to her, in as 'involving' a way as you possibly can. In other words try to make HER feel part of the decision-making to make *and keep* her safe.

- The child must see the doctor. If she cannot be seen straight away, then you must get her to hospital.

- If she becomes unconscious, make sure her airway is clear and she is breathing normally. Put her in the Recovery Position but be prepared to do your ABC Resuscitation Routine if breathing stops.

A for **AIRWAY** (is it clear?)

B for **BREATHING** (is she breathing?)

C for **CIRCULATION** (is her heart beating?)

- Call for an ambulance by dialling 999. Tell them it is urgent and that the child *is in a diabetic coma*.

When a diabetic child becomes unwell at school, *she should never be sent to the medical room on her own.* Please explain this to the teacher. Also make sure you leave your phone number (and your partner/friend/neighbour's telephone number), so that if the child has to be sent home the school is absolutely sure that a responsible person will be there to look after her.

Your child must never be tempted to take any other child's insulin, supposing there were another diabetic child around and she had forgotten hers. It will almost certainly be a different type or dose. *Please warn her about this.*

If a diabetic child is sick, she must always see a doctor.

Please make sure that your child carries some easily recognisable identification to tell those around her that she is a diabetic. An identity

113

necklet or bracelet (like Medic-Alert) is the best. It should be worn at all times, particularly on school outings. Some schools are a bit fussy about 'jewellery' but you must explain to the teacher or Head that this is different, and that the child has to wear it on doctor's orders. Medic-Alert bracelets are not jewellery and could save a child's life.

Diabetics may have all sorts of problems to do with their circulation. If a child with diabetes smokes, the risk of heart disease early in her life is greater. Smoking can also stop the insulin working as well as it should.

You *can't stop* your kids from smoking if they're determined to do so, *but you can* tell them about the risks they take if they do.

If your child has diabetes, or you are looking after a diabetic child, and you need more information, you can write to or phone:

The Youth Department, British Diabetic Association
10 Queen Anne Street, London W1M 0BD.
Tel. 071 323 1531
They produce some excellent pamphlets and have all sorts of back-up services which might help you if you have a diabetic child in the family.

If you want to know more about your child's condition, the following books might help: *So Your Child Has Diabetes?* by Bonnie Estridge and Jo Davies (Vermilion), *If Your Child is Diabetic: An Answer Book for Parents* by Joanne Elliott (Sheldon Press), and *Diabetes: A Young Person's Guide* by Rowan Hillson (Optima).

HYPOGLYCAEMIA – too little sugar (this is the most common reason for a child with diabetes to feel 'funny').

- Reassure and comfort the child.
- If child is conscious *and can swallow*, give her some sweet food urgently – sugar lump, sugary drink, banana. DO NOT send a child who might be 'hypo' anywhere on her own (including the medical room or home).
- If she becomes unconscious, make sure her airway is clear.
- Roll her into the Recovery Position.
- *She needs special medical help urgently.* Call for the ambulance by dialling 999. DON'T WAIT. Tell them the child is in a DIABETIC COMA and *is probably hypoglycaemic*.

THINK

- Have you managed to get some help? Try shouting out of the window or front door.
- Have you called the ambulance? Try to get someone to do this for you.

HYPERGLYCAEMIA – too much sugar.

- Ask the child if she has taken her insulin injection.
- Ask if she has had extra food which might have upset her.
- If she becomes unconscious, make sure her airway is clear.
- Put her in the Recovery Position.
- Ring for an ambulance by dialling 999. Tell them that the child is in a DIABETIC COMA.

12 DIARRHOEA AND VOMITING

BABIES

Diarrhoea and vomiting in a baby is particularly dangerous and should never be ignored. Children cannot cope with a sudden, dramatic loss of fluid because, unlike adults, they cannot replace it quickly and their bodies become dangerously dehydrated (dehydrate means to lose water).

Babies who are breast-fed tend to be less likely to get serious gut infections such as gastro-enteritis, because the breast milk is thought to protect the gut from infection. So if you are bottle feeding, you have to be especially careful about keeping bottles, bottle teats and feeding cups clean and as untouched by human hands as possible. If your baby starts to have diarrhoea and is sick more than once, then *take her off milk* unless she is being breast-fed (in which case keep feeding her, if she wants it), but give her some *cooled*, boiled water from a bottle as well. If she keeps vomiting stop feeding her and just try giving her small amounts of *cooled*, boiled water.

WHAT TO LOOK FOR

- You can usually tell if it is gastro-enteritis because the stools the baby passes are greenish, watery and smelly – they may also have some mucus (clear, sticky stuff) in them. However, the stools may not always look like this – they may just be watery.

- The urine on her nappy may be 'strong' and smelly; this is because the body is trying to hang on to as much fluid as possible, so the waste products that are being passed are not as diluted as they would normally be.

  Be careful to check whether it is urine or watery diarrhoea – it is easy to confuse the two. One of the first things the doctor will ask you is how often she has a 'wet' nappy – and it is important for you to know what it is wet with.

- She will look 'dry' – her mouth and tongue may be parched-looking, her eyes may be glazed, the soft spot at the top of her head may be sunken.

- She will probably be irritable and will not be easily comforted by you.

- Babies often bring their legs up to their chest in pain when they fill their nappy. However, they may not have any pain.

WHAT TO DO

- You must get her to your doctor urgently. If it is the middle of the night, either phone the emergency doctor or, if the baby is still vomiting and having diarrhoea, call the ambulance by dialling 999. Tell them your baby has severe vomiting and diarrhoea.

Very occasionally there is a different reason for vomiting (particularly) and diarrhoea, other than infection. One of these is caused by a thickening of the 'pylorus' (the outlet of the stomach). This narrows so much that most of the food never gets out of the stomach and there is a build-up in the stomach. This is called pyloric stenosis.

This usually happens to boys rather than girls and starts when he is about six weeks old. He will start to be sick in a very startling way – he literally forces the vomit out, almost across the room. The doctor will send him to hospital to have some tests to make sure that it IS his pylorus which is causing the problem. If it is, then he will need to have a small operation. This is highly successful and the child quickly gets back to normal.

CHILDREN

Children with vomiting and diarrhoea, for whatever reason, generally feel unwell and are often in a lot of pain, especially if the gut is swollen and inflamed.

WHAT TO DO

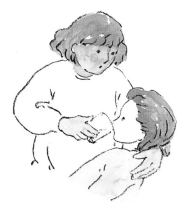

- If a child, no matter what age, gets vomiting and diarrhoea, *take her off food* immediately. It is all right for a child not to eat for a few days, *as long as she drinks*. Some parents and carers may think that children need to eat *something* if they are ill. They don't. The best thing is for them to give their stomach (and therefore their gut) a rest. But it is IMPORTANT that they drink lots of clear fluids – water, maybe flavoured with a drop of squash. (Remember some squashes contain a lot of sugar and this in itself makes an already irritable gut worse.)

- A child with a tummy bug, whatever caused it, is bound to be miserable. There is nothing worse than being sick. It makes the best of us feel awful. Comfort her, keep her hair out of the way and be ready to

117

sponge her down when she has finished. Try not to leave a child on her own when she is being sick, no matter how queasy you may feel – you don't have to look.

We have a 'friendly bucket' (it doesn't have to be a bucket) which is kept specially for being sick in. It's kept in a special place and everyone knows where it is and what it is used for.

ADOLESCENTS

From time to time adolescents make themselves sick. This can be for a variety of complicated reasons that parents may find difficult to understand. The first clue may be that the child starts to lose weight – often a lot of weight. The child may be starving herself or, even more alarming, having alternate periods of starving, bingeing and then making herself sick (bulimia).

She may have a lot of things worrying her which she may not be able to work out without professional help. This combination of problems, which doctors call anorexia (although there are a number of other names which describe it in more detail), should be taken seriously by parents and carers.

You must not pretend to yourself that 'it is only a phase' that children go through – *most children don't*. There are also knock-on effects. If she is in deadly earnest about losing weight – whatever the cost – she may be taking laxatives as well as making herself sick and the combined loss of fluids can be enough to damage her kidneys. If she continues to lose more than a certain amount of her body weight, her periods could also stop.

The giving of food from one person to another is one of the most basic human instincts. 'Society' expects that from babyhood onwards the parent will give and the child will take. If you think that she is vomiting food on a regular basis, or she has lost a lot of weight while she is being 'cared for', it will only be natural for you to feel hurt and rejected. This, however, will complicate the worries and fears you have for the child and the communication between you may get log-jammed because of the raw emotions involved. All of this needs to be sorted out.

WHAT TO DO

Once your child is old enough to make decisions for herself – even if you think she is making the wrong ones about food – let her decide about what, where and how she eats. Some parents just cannot 'let go' and the situation goes from bad to worse. Some of these problems start with the parents not being able to see that the child *is* capable of making sensible decisions and not recognising that she is growing up.

The 'child' may see things differently and may use food as the only weapon she has to make her point of view felt, such as, 'I am an independent person and I can do (and certainly *eat*) what I like.'

Try not to leave the problem until you are both well dug-in. If you are not having much success talking to your child about her eating, which is quite usual (the child may deny there is anything unusual going on and tell you it is all in your imagination), you may want to go and see your GP or Health Visitor to talk it through. They may suggest you see a special counsellor or your doctor may want to refer your child to hospital for an assessment. Don't try to deal with this by yourself. There are people available who are willing and *trained* to help you.

Always phone your doctor if your child is being sick, whatever the cause. If her condition is worrying you, your doctor won't mind being contacted. If he does, you might want to think about changing your doctor.

Be aware that occasionally diarrhoea and particularly vomiting can be a sign of other illnesses. If your child has severe tummy ache as well, it could either be that the gut is sore and inflamed, as you might expect in gastro-enteritis (tummy bug), or it could be that the child has appendicitis (this is a condition where the appendix becomes inflamed and, if it is not dealt with urgently, the child can become seriously ill or even die). As a parent you won't know which it is, but the rule is that *any* diarrhoea and vomiting that goes on for more than twenty-four hours (less in little ones), especially if it is accompanied by bad tummy ache, should always be seen by a doctor.

If you feel that your child is eating too little, 'bingeing' enough to make herself sick, or using food as some other tool to interfere with the relationship between you, then you may want to contact the Eating Disorders Association. This is a network of locally based, country-wide, self-help groups who send out information about the treatment for anorexia nervosa and bulimia, both eating disorders affecting young people. They will also send parents and carers a set of guidelines for coping with children suffering in this way. The address is:

The Eating Disorders Association
Sackville Place, 44-48 Magdalen Street, Norwich, Norfolk NR3 1JU.
Tel. 0603 621414
They are open Monday to Friday 9 a.m. to 6.30 p.m.

The Eating Disorders Association has a lot of reading material to help parents and carers learn more about these distressing conditions. They recommend the following book: *Anorexia Nervosa: Let Me Be* by Professor Arthur Crisp.

You can also phone the Eating Disorders Association for help or advice on:

Helpline 0603 765050 open Monday to Friday between 9 a.m. to 6.30 p.m. OR **Youth Helpline** 0603 765050 open Monday to Wednesday between 4 p.m. and 6 p.m.

119

13 DROWNING

Around twenty-three children drown *around the home* every year, in the bath or garden pond. Out of those, twenty are aged under five. Even children who can swim are not necessarily protected. The fact that a child can swim tends to make parents and carers feel they can relax more than perhaps they should because they *think* that their child would be able to cope if he fell into water. BUT most children learn to swim in a water temperature of between 22°C and 28°C (72°F and 82°F) in their swimming costumes. When a child falls into water accidentally, he will probably be fully clothed and it is usually cold or freezing – and the cold literally takes his breath away. So often the fact of whether or not he can swim is not the point.

Many children are now having some swimming lessons with their clothes on, so if they do get into difficulty, they know what it feels like to be in the water fully clothed. But this doesn't get over the problem of the icy water.

Children, especially babies and toddlers, can drown in the smallest amount of water. Ian, a lively baby of twelve months, crawled over to where his mother had been washing the floor and tipped head first into the bucket. His mother had just gone to answer the doorbell. When she came back he was dead.

NEVER LEAVE AN OLDER CHILD LOOKING AFTER A BABY OR TODDLER IN THE BATH. If her attention wanders for a minute, the little one may slip noiselessly under the water and she may not even have noticed. It simply isn't fair to load a child with that sort of responsibility. Better to miss the bath that night altogether!

So children are not always out of danger in the 'safety' of their own home. Very young children have no idea of danger at all. In fact, never feel that your child is completely safe from having a drowning accident when there is any collection of water (including in wheelbarrows, un-covered dustbins and water-butts) unless you are watching all the time. ROSPA's (The Royal Society for the Prevention of Accidents) advice is that the only way to make garden ponds safe is to turn them into sand-pits until the children are older. DO NOT allow children to wander unsupervised around a neighbour's garden where there is an open pond. It isn't naughtiness when he falls in, it is simply that he does not – cannot – understand.

(The biggest cause of death in children in the USA and Australia is from youngsters falling into friends' or neighbours' swimming pools, or taking a dip in these pools while the owners are out at work or on holiday.)

Keep a special eye on children who enjoy water and are not afraid of it. In many ways they are *more at risk* than the ones who hate swimming.

NEVER in any circumstance push your baby or young child under the water, either to get him 'used' to the water or because you think it will help him learn to swim. While some local authorities encourage these ideas as a 'good thing', there are a number of drownings every year among the under two-year-olds, whose parents or swimming teachers are doing this. So please remember children are NOT 'born swimmers'.

When a child drowns, a number of things happen. When the water hits the back of the throat the muscles seize up and go into spasm. This immediately cuts down the amount of air and therefore oxygen that can get into the lungs. It is the lack of oxygen, rather than the amount of water in the lungs, that will cause the child to die.

The child will also swallow water. If he stays in the water after he becomes unconscious the epiglottis, which normally stops things going down 'the wrong way' (see Chapter 2 on How the Body Works), will relax and water will spill over into the lungs.

WHAT TO DO

● Pull the child out of the water as quickly as you can. If he has fallen into a small bucket or a pond, you will find this fairly easy to do. If, however, he has got into difficulties in a swimming pool or in the sea and you can't swim DO NOT get into the water yourself, you will only get into more difficulty.

● You must SHOUT FOR HELP urgently. If your child has fallen in an out-of-the-way pond or in the sea, people around you may just not realise there is an emergency and think you are larking about. If people come to help, organise them quickly either to form a human chain to pull the child out, or to swim out to him for you. Tell one of them to go and call for an ambulance by dialling 999. Tell them to explain to the ambulance service what has happened and to give precise directions as to how to find you.

● If there is no one to help you, however, even though you know it may not be sensible, you will probably try to save the child yourself. Try to reach him with a pole or a rope if you can. Do not swim if you can wade. If possible take some kind of float with you – it will make the rescue easier. It is vital that before you enter the water you have attracted attention, if this is possible.

● Remember, trying to lift a child out of the water when you are by yourself can be very difficult especially if you are in the water as well.

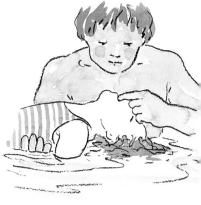

● Quickly LOOK IN HIS MOUTH when you reach him, to see if there is anything blocking his airway, for instance sea-weed, pond-weed, vomit, mud or even a sweet he may have been sucking when he went under water. (Never allow children to chew gum or suck sweets while they swim: it is very dangerous.)

121

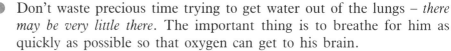

Open his airway (you can do this even though you may be in the water).

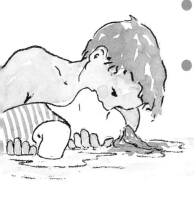

- Don't waste precious time trying to get water out of the lungs – *there may be very little there.* The important thing is to breathe for him as quickly as possible so that oxygen can get to his brain.

- Start mouth-to-mouth (or mouth-to-mouth-and-nose if he is little) breathing as soon as you can. If you are in deep water and cannot stand up, you may be able to give him an occasional breath while you are towing him ashore – this is extremely difficult and training and practice would help (check with your local swimming pool for life saving courses).

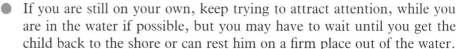

  When you can stand up in the water use one arm to support the child's body and your other hand to support his head. Hold his nose if you are doing mouth-to-mouth breathing. If the child is little it may be easier to breathe into his mouth and nose at the same time.

- If you are still on your own, keep trying to attract attention, while you are in the water if possible, but you may have to wait until you get the child back to the shore or can rest him on a firm place out of the water.

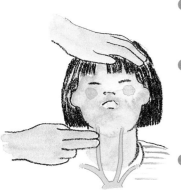

Feeling for the neck pulse (carotid).

- Check that someone has called for an ambulance by dialling 999. If you are in a neighbour's garden or in the swimming pool you may have done this already. But if no one has told you the ambulance is coming, *always check.* Most people, no matter how well-meaning they are, just watch and do nothing.

- Check his circulation by taking his pulse. If his pulse is all right then continue breathing for him until the child breathes for himself or help arrives.

- REMEMBER you cannot tell for some time how good – or bad – a recovery the child will make after this kind of accident. Often a child who has been in very cold water has a better chance than a child in a 'warm' swimming pool. The lungs may collapse quickly or slowly, the brain may be able to survive or not. Keep on trying to get his breathing started until you can get him to hospital.

Feeling for the arm pulse in a baby (brachial).

- Keep checking his pulse at frequent intervals and if his heart stops, start resuscitation immediately to try and start it again. PRESS FIVE TIMES and then give ONE BREATH. Do not give up until medical help arrives or you get him to hospital.

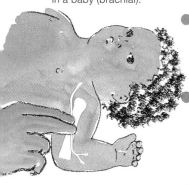

- If, at any time, he starts breathing by himself and his heart is beating, roll him over into the Recovery Position. The chances are that as soon as he starts to breathe he will be sick because he has swallowed so much water. Rolling him into the Recovery Position will stop him inhaling the vomit into his lungs.

- Reassure him that he is all right and talk calmly to him. Even though he may not seem to hear you he will be comforted by your voice.

● Keep him as warm as you can by putting a blanket underneath him. If you can, towel him dry and put two or three *light* blankets, towels or clothes over the top of him. Don't be tempted to warm him up too quickly (see Chapter 21 on Hypothermia and Hyperthermia).

● DO NOT give him anything to eat or drink.

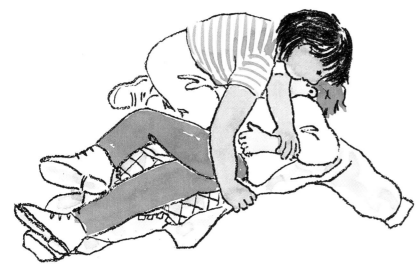

● ALL CHILDREN who have had any kind of drowning accident MUST BE TAKEN TO HOSPITAL.

Remember, do not leave children alone in the bath and always have a responsible adult swimmer to supervise them when they go swimming.

Pull the child out of the water. DO NOT *waste time trying to get water out of the lungs – there may be very little there.*

THINK

● Have you managed to get some help? Try shouting to attract attention.
● Have you called the ambulance? Try to get someone to do this for you.
● Have you checked for DANGER?

IF he is unconscious, start your ABC RESUSCITATION ROUTINE as soon as you can. (You may be able to give a few breaths to him while you are in the water – although this may be difficult to do.)

Now check 'A' for AIRWAY – is it clear?

IF HE DOESN'T RESPOND: OPEN THE AIRWAY. Tilt the child's head back and lift his chin forward. REMEMBER babies' necks are chubbier and more fragile. **Be gentle yet firm enough to tilt head back so airway is open.**

Now check 'B' for BREATHING

LOOK
LISTEN } for breathing
FEEL

IF THE CHILD IS NOT BREATHING: BREATHE FOR THE CHILD. Cover his mouth, or nose and mouth, with your mouth. Give him FIVE separate breaths. Watch his chest rise with each breath. REMEMBER you need *less* breath for babies.

Now check 'C' for CIRCULATION

Is his heart beating? Check for the pulse. Feel the neck (or arm in a baby) for a pulse. **If there is no pulse and you haven't got help GET IT NOW.**

IF YOU CANNOT FEEL A PULSE: DO CHEST COMPRESSION. Feel for the right place – one finger-breadth below the nipple line. Press on the chest, at a rate of **100 presses per minute.**

For children over one year old: Use the 'heel' of one hand only, with your arm straight. **Press fifteen times to every two breaths** (so your hand presses in about 2.5-3.5cm or 1-1½ inches each time).

For babies: Use two fingers only and **press five times to one breath** (so your fingers press in about 2cm which is about ¾ of an inch each time).

KEEP DOING THIS UNTIL THE AMBULANCE ARRIVES.

DRUG ABUSE, SOLVENT SNIFFING AND ALCOHOL

14

Children who take drugs can be any age. I have referred to them in this chapter as children, even though some of them may be young adults.

The reasons why children take drugs or sniff substances are complicated. It may be because they are lonely and they feel that sniffing (for instance) will give them more confidence and make them 'part of the crowd'. There is often a tremendous amount of group pressure to do what everyone *thinks* everyone else is doing.

It is impossible to give a breakdown in this book of all the drugs that are around, or to describe the individual effects of each drug. (There are a number of very good publications which do this; see page 137.) It is important, however, for you to find out as much as you can about the drugs that are around in your area BEFORE there is a crisis in your house, and to talk openly about their dangers to your child. There may never be a crisis, but at least you will know what your child might get up to and be comforted that she will probably cope better with some background information if she is offered any drugs.

Parents may argue that the only answer to any sort of drugs that children are offered is for them to SAY NO, but this does not take into account the need that many children have to experiment with other sensations. 'After all,' Andy Horne, Director of Westminster Drug Project suggests, 'that's what drives a child to twirl herself round and round until she makes herself dizzy, not once but over and over again – not because it's pleasant, but because it gives her a different experience to the one that she knows – a buzz – that's what drug-taking is all about.'

You may think that as a good parent, you will be able to persuade your child not to take drugs. But be aware of the tremendous influence of friends and other children in and out of school. This is a force to be reckoned with. Children are often scared to say 'no' because of this pressure and because of the need to be 'one of the crowd'. So the message you could give to your child is: you CAN say 'no' *if you want to.*

There are other factors which parents might bear in mind that can influence whether or not a child takes the plunge into drugs.

Adolescence itself is a mystery to many adults. Maybe the whole process was so awful for them that when they are older they forget or can no longer identify with some of the problems. In the same way some children sail through it all without a sulk, spot, or sexual fantasy. Others get the lot, together! But please don't fall into the trap of confusing a rather stormy adolescence with other things that you think might be going on, such as taking drugs.

If a child comes from a disturbed, violent or unloved background or she has emotional problems that are not being dealt with, she might be more likely to turn to some kind of alternative comfort, such as sex or drugs, to take her out of herself.

Adults – even parents – looking after children may leave old bottles of pills which are not used up lying around the home. These may be dangerous drugs from the doctor or just aspirin or cough mixture. Whatever they are, it is common sense to lock them up. These drugs are just asking to be tried by bored or curious youngsters. Little children may also think they are sweets.

DRUGS

Drug-taking and experimenting is part of the nineties youth culture. This is a difficult fact for parents to accept, but unless it is faced there will be little chance of communicating with children about drugs, let alone helping them if they really get into trouble. Some children get into a mess with drugs: for example at least two children a week die from sniffing a substance of some sort.

Drugs are around everywhere and many children will experiment with them at some time in their lives – even YOURS! However, the picture of the pusher loitering at the school gate waiting to pounce on some poor unsuspecting child is largely not true. Many social gatherings will have some drugs being passed around to share – but to put it into some kind of perspective, the two drugs that cause the most damage to health in Britain today are tobacco and alcohol. I am not suggesting that you shouldn't worry if you feel your child is 'on' something, but there are obviously some drugs that should be of more concern than others. The important thing is that your child is aware of the dangers of what she is taking.

Ecstasy

The best advice to a child is *to know what you are taking* and *know roughly what effect it is going to have on you*. Ecstasy is a 'designer drug' and she will never know exactly what is in each tablet. It is already causing a lot of concern because it is thought to have severe side-effects and has caused a number of sudden deaths (even for first-time users).

Barbiturates

Barbiturates are dangerous and if mixed with other drugs, particularly alcohol, they are deadly. (In the 1970s many children died for this reason.) Children who become addicted to barbiturates really need expert medical help because the drugs disturb all of the body's normal functions including sleep, appetite and, for girls, their periods (which may stop altogether).

Cannabis

This drug is normally smoked and is thought by many of those working in the drug field to be much safer than alcohol or even nicotine, unless it is very heavily used (Queen Victoria is said to have used it for her period pains). If, however, it is used by people who have some sort of physical or mental illness – such as diabetes (see Chapter 11 on Diabetes) or schizophrenia – they can become destabilised – that is, their treatment can be knocked off-course by taking drugs that haven't been prescribed by a doctor.

'Special K'

The latest drug of abuse at the time of writing is 'special K'. Doctors know this drug as ketamine. It is used as an anaesthetic in hospitals or in extreme emergencies on the battlefield. However, hospitals tend not to use it now because of the terrible nightmares the patients experience when coming round from the anaesthetic.

The drug is extremely dangerous as it causes hallucinations, and separates the mind from the body so that children who take it have no idea that they are hallucinating. It is sold on the street in tablet form which can be swallowed, or crushed and sniffed. As ketamine is an anaesthetic, it will cause unconsciousness. If this happens, put the child gently into the Recovery Position, telling her what you are doing. (Remember an 'unconscious' child can lapse in and out of consciousness and hearing your voice will comfort her.) Make sure her airway is open and check her breathing and if it stops, start your ABC Resuscitation Routine.

A for **AIRWAY**   (is it clear?)

B for **BREATHING**   (is she breathing?)

C for **CIRCULATION**   (is her heart beating?)

SOLVENTS

Solvents can be dangerous, depending on *what* is sniffed and *how* it is sniffed. Children are sniffing all sorts of peculiar things, from paint sprays and cleaning agents to nail-polish remover and anything in between. The main danger is that many of these substances are very close to anaesthetic agents and can cause unconsciousness.

127

There are lots of things that a child who is even thinking about sniffing should know about – but this is a difficult situation for parents to deal with. If parents tell their child how to sniff 'safely' it looks as if they are encouraging her to do it, but if they don't tell her, she could die. (The Institute for the Study of Drug Dependence, ISDD, has produced some excellent leaflets which will help you and your child know what to do about solvents – see page 137 for their address.)

There is a small risk of something called 'sudden sniffing death' if a child who has been sniffing solvents suddenly does a lot of exercise or is chased by someone. *It is very rare* but you might want to be aware of this.

These are some of the most dangerous solvents:

Gas lighter fuel

This solvent 'cools' the tissues at the back of the throat and they swell up, causing the child to suffocate. (Try to imagine what it feels like if you spill lighter fuel on the back of your hand; well, this is what happens to the throat.) Inhaling gas lighter fuel is one of the causes of sudden death.

Aerosols

Sprayed into the throat, and therefore directly into the lungs, aerosols by-pass the normal protective breathing mechanism which filters out harmful bits and pieces in the air we normally breathe in. The lungs can just seize up and the child stops breathing.

WHAT TO LOOK FOR

You might suspect a child has taken drugs or solvents if:

● The child's behaviour becomes aggressive or totally withdrawn. She may be holed up for days in her room – or worse, walking the streets, looking as if she is drunk, agitated, or confused about the time of day or night. She may have symptoms of paranoia – feeling that people are out to get her – or she may have a high level of anxiety or be depressed.

● Your child could have an unusual amount of energy – and would dance her socks off, given the chance – but she will then be totally exhausted and will probably sleep for the whole of the following day.

● You may find money missing – a drug habit is expensive (although solvents are cheap).

● You may find various bits of 'equipment' such as small pieces of cardboard, scorched knives or tin-foil, sticky crisp-bags or polythene bags, and of course traces of powder or tablets in her room or where she has been with friends. Be careful, however, before jumping to conclusions – there could be some very simple explanation.

● You might smell what you think are solvents on your child (they stink!) or find sticky stuff on her sweater that refuses to come out in the wash. You may notice peculiar marks on her sleeves – some children sniff correction fluid thinner from their shirt cuffs.

● You may find out that your child has been taking time off school. This may have nothing to do with drugs at all, but just to do with wanting to buck the system. But it may be that a group of children have been meeting to take drugs. The time to worry is when your child is doing this by herself. Children are in much more danger if they smoke, sniff, swallow or inject drugs *alone*. This is rare but it generally means that they have other problems and they are much more seriously into drugs. If they do take drugs on their own and things go wrong there is no one to get help.

NOTE: If your child has epilepsy or diabetes, you might think something is wrong (it *could* be drugs) if she suddenly becomes destabilised – in other words, if a child with epilepsy starts to fit again (see Chapter 17 on Fits) or if an adolescent with diabetes starts to become 'hypo' or even goes into a coma (see Chapter 11 on Diabetes).

WHAT TO DO

● This may have been going on a long time or *it may be the first time* your child has tried drugs. She may just be trying to challenge authority and, like it or not, YOU are authority! If you blow it, you could push her into an even more difficult situation – for both of you. You need to handle it carefully, sensibly and sensitively.

● The first thing to do is to arm yourself with as much information as possible. Find out the street names of the drugs (what she calls them) so that you are both talking the same language. Don't pooh-pooh this idea, it may be all you have to help you communicate with her.

● *Get to know the dangers* of the drug you think your child is into and try to bring these into the discussion, rather than taking the immediate 'don't ever touch it again' approach. Tackling it this way takes courage but in the end it could save your child a lot of heartache – it may even save her life. You may also want to find out what happens if she overdoses (ODs) on whatever it is she is taking. You need to know what to do if there is ever an emergency.

● Don't immediately feel that you cannot cope. If you have an open, honest relationship with your child then you are probably as good as anyone else at dealing with it, *as long as you know what you are talking about*. So find out the facts.

● If you haven't got an open, honest relationship now could be the time to try to start having one. Or maybe your child just needs MORE of you, more of your time, more of your emotional energy. Maybe you thought she didn't need you, and maybe *she* thought she didn't either . . .

But perhaps the relationship between you isn't that good. You have to face the fact, painful though it may be, that you can't talk to each other at the moment. If this is the case and you feel your child needs help, try to point her in the direction of someone she can talk to and who will listen to her. If she feels she can't talk to anyone she knows, SCODA (details on page 137) will be able to give your child information on where to get help in your area.

EMERGENCY TREATMENT

There is little more scary than seeing your child in what is generally called a 'drug-induced crisis'. In other words, she has taken an overdose of a drug and is now extremely ill, either mentally or physically.

There is an amazing amount of wrong and sometimes dangerous information flying around the drug scene. Drug users and helpers sometimes find it difficult to sort out the fact from the fiction.

There are a number of states a child might be in after she has taken drugs. She may be:

- Tense and panicky.

- Conscious but drowsy.

- Unconscious.

All of these need careful handling.

WHAT TO DO

When you find her

- Keep calm. If this is your child's first experience of a drug crisis she will be terrified (for all sorts of reasons, but made worse by the fact that you have found out). This is not the time to start ranting and raving at her, no matter how tempted you might be! Try to find out what happened:

- *What drug*. How much has she taken? See if there is anything lying about that can give you a clue: bottles, syringes, foil, plastic bags.

- *In what way*. By mouth, injection, or by sniffing.

- *How long ago. Try to find out* from her or her friends when she last took anything. (They will all be terrified of saying anything.)

- *Anything else*. Might she also have been drinking alcohol, or have taken a variety of drugs?

● *Has she been in an accident*, is she injured, has she got diabetes? (See Chapter 11 on Diabetes.)

● She may, however, be in another state and you should be aware of it. She may be 'having the time of her life' and will be giggling, talkative, energetic and thoroughly enjoying herself, with no 'bad' effects at all. In this case leave her until the effect wears off and talk to her at some time when you think it is good for both of you, when you feel she might listen to you.

If she is tense and panicky

Some drugs give the child a feeling of extreme panic or make her have short spells of 'psychosis'. Psychosis is a mental state where the person is not in touch with reality (out of her head). She may think someone wants to kill her, or she may hear voices telling her to do some evil deed. She may think she is God and can do things woman couldn't normally do, like fly, or walk on water or across a parapet. Many young people have died in this way, not from the drugs themselves but *from what the drugs have made them think they can do.*

● You must calm and reassure her. This child might be terrified, especially if this is the first time she has had this experience.

● Move her away from onlookers, or just tell those around her to go away, quickly and quietly. The more people there are around, the more frantic she may become.

● Talk to her quietly. To hear your voice will calm her as long as you are not laying into her about the dangers or stupidity of taking drugs.

● Keep noise and light levels down. If she is very agitated, she may be saying terrible things about you. Try not to turn it into a slanging match – ignore what she is saying and keep talking calmly and sensibly. Don't overdo the sympathy at this stage – even if you feel it!

● If she is overbreathing (almost panting or gasping), she may experience numbness and tingling of her fingers and toes. She may feel dizzy and sick or she may vomit. Talk firmly to her – tell her what she is doing and that you want her to breathe like this. Get her to follow you in a regular slow breathing pattern (count to three on the in-breath and again to three on the out-breath).

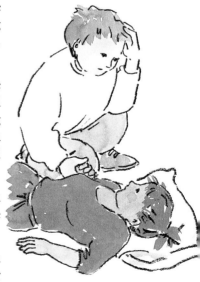

● Hold her hand if she'll let you, even cuddle her (but only if you are a cuddly family – if not she may think you are going to attack her). If she does lash out at you, don't hit her back.

● Don't try to restrain her if she becomes violent, just turn away from her, but if possible don't go out of the room. Carry on talking to her calmly and without emotion.

This period might last two or three hours, or more. You will have to be

131

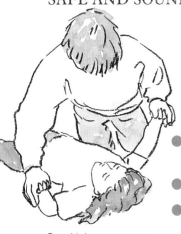

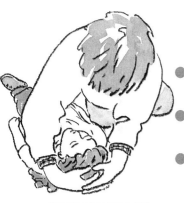

Go with her movements.

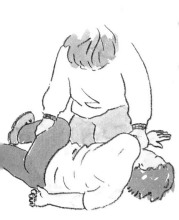

Cushion her head with your hands.

patient, but in this time the panic and feelings of persecution *will* lessen and she will be able to talk reasonably to you. Try to leave the 'deep and meaningful' chat to some other time, when you have all had a chance to calm down.

There is a possibility that she might fit (see Chapter 17 on Fits). This is what will happen if she does:

- Her muscles will start to twitch and her arms and legs will make odd jerking movements.

- Her eyes may roll backwards into her head.

- There may be some stiffness or arching of her back, as the head is pushed backwards. Or she may just thrash about. She may hold her breath.

- She may go blue and the veins in her face and neck may stand out.

- She may froth at the mouth.

Once a fit has started there is nothing you can do to stop it – it has a life of its own. So although it is a bit scary to watch her 'out of contact', the only thing you can do at this stage is to keep her safe.

- Don't try to stop any thrashing movements but you can lie next to her and 'go with' her movements to prevent her injuring herself.

- Move away any hard objects that she might strike herself on while she is thrashing around on the floor.

- Cushion her head with your hands or forearms, but DON'T prevent any movements – in other words, just go with her movements, trying to protect her as much as possible.

- DON'T put anything between her teeth. (This is now considered to be extremely dangerous – she could bite and break whatever it is you have stuck in her mouth and inhale the broken bit. Alternatively, she could break her teeth, which she won't thank you for later on in life.)

- DON'T try to move her during the fit, unless she is a danger to herself or to other people.

- As soon as the fit is over, roll her into the Recovery Position. Make sure her airway is open and that she is breathing easily.

- Comfort and soothe her. She may drift in and out of sleep at this stage and will certainly be feeling groggy, but hearing your voice will calm her.

- Stay with her, or near her, until she is fully recovered.

- If you haven't done so already, send for an ambulance by dialling 999 and tell them what has happened.

● If the child fits for a long time there is a chance that she could stop breathing. This is very rare, but be prepared to carry out your ABC Resuscitation Routine.

> **A** for **AIRWAY** (is it clear?)
>
> **B** for **BREATHING** (is she breathing?)
>
> **C** for **CIRCULATION** (is her heart beating?)

If she is conscious but drowsy

Some drugs will make her more drowsy than others. She may even begin to lose consciousness – even if it is only for a moment. Drug overdoses make the body act as if it has been poisoned – and it has been. If the child doesn't lose consciousness she will have enormous out-pourings of spit usually followed by retching, vomiting and bad tummy ache.

● Try to find out what happened (see above).

● If she vomits, make sure that she is not lying on her back, in case she inhales it. If she is losing consciousness and she starts to be sick, roll her over into the Recovery Position.

● If she has stomach cramps, she may become very shocked. Treat her for shock. (See Chapter 27 on Shock.)

> ### REMEMBER – SHOCK LOOKS LIKE THIS
>
> ● Her face may be very pale and grey-looking
>
> ● Her skin may feel cold and clammy
>
> ● Her pulse may feel fast and weak
>
> ● She may be frightened and fidgety
>
> ● She may be very thirsty
>
> ● She may yawn and 'gasp' for air
>
> ● She may say everything feels fuzzy
>
> ● She may become unconscious

● You must calm and reassure her. She will be embarrassed and frightened, especially if this is the first time she has had this experience – but each time is probably as terrifying as the last.

● Move her away from onlookers, or just tell those around her to go away, quickly and quietly. The more people there are around, the more embarrassed and agitated she will become.

● Talk to her quietly; just to hear your voice will calm her as long as you are not choosing this moment to tell her what a total idiot she is! (She knows that already.)

● Keep noise and light levels down. Don't overdo the sympathy at this stage.

● If she begins to lose consciousness, open her airway and check her breathing. If it stops, start your ABC Resuscitation Routine.

> **A** for **AIRWAY** (is it clear?)
>
> **B** for **BREATHING** (is she breathing?)
>
> **C** for **CIRCULATION** (is her heart beating?)

If she is breathing normally roll her over into the Recovery Position.

● You need to get her to hospital before her condition gets worse. Get someone to call for an ambulance by dialling 999.

If she is unconscious

Once a child who has taken an overdose of drugs loses consciousness and cannot be roused, you must get medical help, even though the hospital might start asking questions that she (or you) might not want to answer. The police are not normally informed of illegal drug use, but ISDD (the Institute for the Study of Drug Dependence) say even if they are, 'It's better to be alive and in trouble, than dead and safe from arrest!'

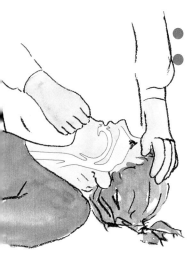

● Call an ambulance by dialling 999 and tell them what has happened.

● *Meanwhile watch this child carefully.* Children who have taken an overdose of drugs to the extent that they have become unconscious may go downhill rapidly. If breathing stops, open her airway and start your ABC Resuscitation Routine.

> **A** for **AIRWAY** (is it clear?)
>
> **B** for **BREATHING** (is she breathing?)
>
> **C** for **CIRCULATION** (is her heart beating?)

Be careful: normally you would take her pulse at the neck (carotid artery). It really is the only place to get an accurate picture of what is going on. Just be aware, though, that a child who has taken a drug overdose, who is still conscious or semi-conscious, may have strong feelings of persecution and any attempt to touch her neck may be misunderstood as an attempt to harm her – even by her own parent. It is just a case of being aware of this and not 'lunging' at her. When it comes to taking her pulse – like everything else you may do to help her while she is in this state – gently explain to her what you are going to do.

Never assume that a child who is unconscious can't hear you. She may lapse in and out of consciousness to find you doing things to her that might frighten her and make the situation worse.

- Open her *airway* and check that it doesn't get kinked again as she moves around. (Just because she is unconscious doesn't mean that she will always lie still.)

- Make sure her *breathing* is not being stopped by any obstruction such as a blocked-up nose, or from her airway being kinked.

- Look in her *mouth* to see if there is anything blocking her airway, such as a piece of food, or vomit. (There might be clues to this around the place you found her.) Do a quick 'finger-sweep' to double check there is nothing in the mouth.

- Loosen any *tight clothing* either at her neck or waist. This will help her to breathe more easily.

- *If, at any time, you feel uneasy about her breathing* WHETHER SHE HAS INJURIES OR NOT (maybe she is making a breathing noise, as if something is stuck in her throat), put her in the Recovery Position, so that if she vomits there is less chance that she will inhale it and block her airway. If you have a blanket or warm coat to hand, you may like to roll it under her.

- Check to see if there is any obvious serious injury, such as bleeding or fractures (see Chapter 6 on Bleeding and Chapter 18 on Fractures and Bone Injuries).

- Stay with the child at all times until the ambulance arrives. Check her breathing and pulse at about five-minute intervals.

- NEVER try to give an unconscious child anything to eat or drink – *not even the smallest sip of water* – she will choke.

ALWAYS call for medical help and don't worry that the drugs your child has taken might be illegal. The doctor's or hospital's main concern is to make the child well again and they are rarely interested in involving the police.

If a child is found in the street or a public place, having passed out and looking as if she might have taken drugs, and is found by the police, they will get the child to hospital but they will probably want to interview her at a later date. They will want to do this sympathetically and, if possible, with the support of the family.

ALCOHOL

Every year about 1000 under-fifteen-year-olds are admitted to hospital suffering from alcohol poisoning. Some of these have been accidentally poisoned when alcohol has been left around the home – this may be a half-finished glass of something that looks like water, such as gin or vodka, or the child may have got hold of a bottle and been able to un-screw the top and take a swig. This is particularly likely if the parent does this from time to time. So watch it – if you do take the occasional swig from the bottle – don't let the kids see you do it!

Children see people drinking alcohol in many situations, so they see the good effects it has on adults, and the bad. They may even *feel* the bad effects themselves if an already depressed parent drinks too much and takes their anger and frustration out on the child.

Adults are often persuaded against their better judgement to 'have another quick one'. Imagine then, how difficult it is for a teenager, just starting to drink and to be 'one of the crowd', to find enough self-confidence to say 'not for me thanks'.

Of course many children don't want to stop when they are on a binge. Once drunk, they are no longer capable of making any sensible decisions, and that is when they start getting into trouble.

Many of these problems might be avoided if you can talk and com-municate with your child about the use (and abuse) of alcohol early enough in her life. Just as with drugs and sex, your child has to have enough self-confidence and self-esteem – she has got to *like* herself enough – not to feel pressurised into doing what she *thinks* everyone else is doing.

Just be aware that if *you* get 'legless' on a regular basis, there is less chance that your child will take your advice very seriously about not drinking too much.

If you are worried that your child or a child you know is drinking on a regular basis, and particularly if she is hiding this from you, there may be a risk she is becoming dependent on alcohol. This can cause brain damage in young people. You may be able to persuade her to go with you to Alcoholics Anonymous (local address in the phone book), an organisation set up to help alcohol-dependent people. Or you may want to contact Al-Anon (local address in the phone book) for relatives of those who have this problem.

The important thing is for you to talk to someone about it – and share the burden. You may want to start with your GP.

If you want further information on drug and solvent abuse, you may want to contact any of the organisations listed below. If you need in-formation on drugs or solvent abuse, contact ISDD. If you want information on drug services and/or support for the family in your area, contact SCODA.

If you want leaflets to learn about what drugs your child might be into, or just for your own interest so that you can be as street-wise as your child but, more important, *know* and *understand* the dangers of specific drug use, contact ISDD. They have an excellent selection of leaflets and a very good library – everyone there really wants to help give out as much information as possible.

ISDD: The Institute for the Study of Drug Dependence
1 Hatton Place, London EC1N 8ND.
Tel. 071 430 1993

SCODA: The Standing Conference on Drug Abuse
(same address as ISDD)
Tel. 071 430 2341

If you want information about solvent abuse, contact RE-SOLV. They also produce lots of pamphlets, have videos for parents, run support groups and publish a newsletter.

RE-SOLV: The Society for the Prevention of Solvent and Volatile Substances Abuse
St Mary's Chambers, 19 Station Road, Stone, Staffordshire ST15 8JP.
Tel. 0785 46097/817885

For twenty-four-hour telephone emergency legal advice and information about anything relating to drugs, particularly if a youngster has been picked up by police for a drugs offence:

RELEASE 071 603 8654.

Freefone 100: Twenty-four-hour service for any drug-related problems. The answerphone will give you the number of your local emergency drugs service. Some of these are run by trained counsellors and some by concerned family-based groups. They can give an enormous amount of support.

For more information about the many different types of drugs that are available 'on the street', you may like to read *Drug Warning* by David Stockley of the Metropolitan Police (Optima). There are also two excellent booklets which you may like to read: *Solvents: A Parent's Guide, The Signs, The Dangers, What to Do* and *Drugs: A Parent's Guide, The Signs, The Dangers, What to Do*. These are available free of charge from:

Health Publications
Unit Heywood Stores, No. 2 Side, Manchester Road, Heywood, Lancashire OL10 2PZ.

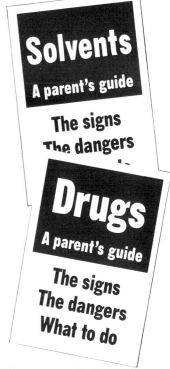

These two excellent leaflets are available from SCODA.

- Move her away from onlookers.
- Talk to her quietly, just hearing your voice will calm her. If she is over-breathing in panic, tell her not to, but to follow the long slow breathing pattern that you will show her.
- Hold her hand if she will let you.
- Keep noise and light levels low.
- If she wants to be sick, roll her into the Recovery Position.
- Ring 999 for ambulance. Tell them exactly what has happened.

IF SHE FITS:
- Once fit starts DO NOT try to stop it, or move the child.
- Loosen any tight clothing round neck and chest.
- Protect child from injury by cushioning her head in your hands. Remove hard objects that are lying near her.
- DON'T put anything between her teeth.
- Once fit is over reassure and *roll into Recovery Position.*
- If child fits for a long time, *she might stop breathing.*

THINK

- Have you got help? Try shouting out of the window or front door.
- Have you called the ambulance? Try to get someone to do this.
- Have you checked for DANGER?
- Shake and shout at the child to see if she is conscious.

IF THE CHILD BECOMES UNCONSCIOUS OR STOPS BREATHING: be ready to start your ABC RESUSCITATION ROUTINE.

Now check   'A' for AIRWAY – is it clear?

IF SHE DOESN'T RESPOND: OPEN THE AIRWAY. Tilt her head back and lift her chin forward.

Now check   'B' for BREATHING

LOOK
LISTEN } for breathing
FEEL

IF THE CHILD IS NOT BREATHING: BREATHE FOR THE CHILD. Cover her mouth with your mouth. Give her five separate breaths. Watch her chest rise with each breath.

Now check   'C' for CIRCULATION

Is her heart beating? Feel the neck for the pulse.

IF YOU CANNOT FEEL A PULSE: DO CHEST COMPRESSION. Feel for the right place – one finger-breadth below the nipple line. Press on the chest, at a rate of **100 presses per minute.** Use the 'heel' of one hand only, with your arm straight. **Press fifteen times to every two breaths** (so your hand presses in about 2.5-3.5cm or 1-1½ inches each time).

ELECTRIC SHOCK

15

Most labour-saving gadgets and equipment in the home are run by electricity and most of them are taken for granted. That is, until children come along. All of a sudden little fingers are poking and exploring things that, if touched in the wrong way or with sticky or wet fingers, can quite simply kill them.

If an electric current goes through a child's body it can cause severe and sometimes fatal injuries. Try to be aware of this and take as many safety precautions as you can – both in terms of effort *and* expense.

Electric currents come from either low- or high-voltage supply, or from lightning. Low-voltage electricity powers all our household appliances (normally 240 volts in the UK).

High-voltage electricity powers overhead pylons and railway lines, and is present in the Electricity Board substations (the ones with DANGER – KEEP OUT written all over them). The electricity in these substations can go up to 400,000 volts.

Electricity entering a child's body can do a number of things:

- The shock can cause the heart to change from beating to quivering like a jelly – this is called fibrillation and it is extremely serious. It stops the blood from being pumped around the body as it should be and the child may die.

- It can cause the heart to stop altogether, if the shock is big enough for that particular child.

- It can burn the child, from the point where the electricity goes into the body, to the point where it leaves micro-seconds later. This can cause serious injury to the internal organs as the electricity zips through the system. There may be serious injuries that you cannot see.

WHAT TO LOOK FOR

- She may be lying on or near some electrical appliance or plug.

- Her face may be white – her breathing and heart may have stopped at the same time.

- She may have deep burns at the point where the electricity entered (and possibly left) her body.

- There may be a 'burnt' smell, of flesh if it is really bad, or of the appliance itself.

- She will almost certainly be in shock – if the electric current was not big enough to make her breathing stop.

● The child's heart may have stopped with the strength of the current – children are more severely affected than adults by sudden-impact injuries like electric shock. In other words, it is more likely to make a child's heart stop than an adult's.

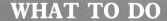

WHAT TO DO

For low-voltage electric shock

These are ones that take place around the home or even in shops or offices.

● DO NOT touch the child UNTIL you have removed her from the electricity supply.

● You need to get her away from the electricity supply without putting yourself in danger. If there is water around you will have to find something to stand on that won't conduct electricity, such as a pile of newspapers, a telephone book, a wooden box, or a rubber or plastic mat, *before* you touch her. The easiest and quickest thing to do is to put on a pair of DRY rubber gloves and pull her away from the supply, by her clothes. (Know where the rubber gloves are: this is almost as important as knowing where the electricity supply is.)

Alternatively, push the child away from the supply with something such as a long-handled wooden brush, a rolled-up newspaper or a *rubber-soled* shoe. Or, if you are desperate, drag her away by her clothing without touching her skin, but remember some clothing made from nylon or man-made fibre conducts electricity.

● Switch off the electricity as soon as you possibly can (if you haven't already) after you have made the child safe, TO PREVENT ANOTHER ACCIDENT.

● DO YOU KNOW WHERE THE MAINS SWITCH IS FOR YOUR ELECTRICITY (OR GAS) SUPPLY? CAN YOU GET TO IT IN AN EMERGENCY?

● REMEMBER, if you turn the electricity off after dark, you will turn the lights off as well. Once they are off you will find it difficult both to deal with the child and to find your way to all the things you will need, such as the telephone. Keep a torch handy for occasions like this.

● REMEMBER, if the child loses consciousness, open her airway and check her breathing.

If you think her heart has stopped, begin your ABC Resuscitation Routine immediately AFTER you have removed her from the electricity supply. (See Chapter 3 on ABC Resuscitation Routine.)

> **A** for **AIRWAY**   (is it clear?)
>
> **B** for **BREATHING**   (is she breathing?)
>
> **C** for **CIRCULATION**   (is her heart beating?)

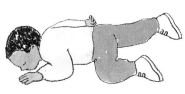

● As soon as she is breathing, roll her over into the Recovery Position.

● Call for an ambulance if you haven't already done so by dialling 999. Tell the ambulance driver anything you can about the type of electric shock and how long you think the child might have been in contact with the electric current (minutes or seconds).

● If the electric shock has not made her breathing or heart stop she will be in shock (see Chapter 27 on Shock).

REMEMBER – SHOCK LOOKS LIKE THIS

● Her face may be very pale and grey-looking

● Her skin may feel cold and clammy

● Her pulse may feel fast and weak

● She may be frightened and fidgety

● She may be very thirsty

● She may yawn and 'gasp' for air

● She may say everything feels fuzzy

● She may become unconscious

Remember a child can be badly shocked by this type of injury and if it isn't treated properly she could die.

● If the child looks as if she is going to vomit, put her in the Recovery Position.

● Constantly reassure her. There is little more terrifying than this sort of injury and she will want to hear your voice and be comforted by it. If she is conscious but too badly hurt to cuddle you, give her a teddy to hold. It might help a little bit.

● Cool any burn with cold water, but *be absolutely sure you have completely removed her from any electricity supply*. Look at the burns carefully – they may be deeper than you think. Look for any other burn marks, where the electricity may have *left* the body (for 'exit' burn see 'Electrical Burns' in Chapter 7 on Burns and Scalds).

● ALL ELECTRICAL BURNS SHOULD BE SEEN URGENTLY IN HOSPITAL.

141

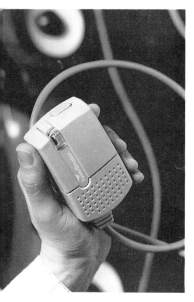

(You may want to think about installing RCDs – Residual Current Devices – on some of your electrical appliances, or on the fuse board itself. RCDs should be installed *in addition to* any other electricity safety devices you may have around the house, like fuses or circuit breakers. They work by 'tripping out' and absorbing a fatal electric shock in milli-seconds so that the RCD takes the brunt of the shock and not the child.)

For high-voltage electric shock

Tragically, there may be very little you can do except call for help. Call the police and ambulance immediately. You can't turn off the electricity supply yourself.

This is an extremely serious and usually fatal accident for any child to have. She will have severe burns from having been in contact with anything up to 400,000 volts, if she survives. This includes overhead cables, railway lines and electricity substations. There is no way that you can touch her, or attempt to rescue her from the immediate area of the accident, *until the electricity supply has been turned off.*

If the ambulance hasn't arrived, do your ABC Resuscitation Routine as soon as you are given the all-clear to go to the child.

A for **AIRWAY**   (is it clear?)

B for **BREATHING**   (is she breathing?)

C for **CIRCULATION**   (is her heart beating?)

If there is no one else around to give the all-clear you want to take the chance that she is not still 'live'. Her heart will almost certainly have stopped, as will her breathing. Your chances of saving her life are slim.

You can only touch her if she has been thrown more than twenty yards (eighteen metres) from where she had the electric shock – this is a safe enough distance from the source of the electricity for you to touch her without being electrocuted yourself. You *may* also be able to go near her – though you will never be able to tell for sure – if she has fallen BELOW the electricity supply. For example, if the child has climbed a telegraph pole to try to get something down from the overhead cables the shock may knock her off the pole to the ground below.

The same sort of injury can happen if a child climbs or falls onto railway lines. There are two sorts of railway lines. One has a live rail *on the track itself* (the 'conductor' line runs alongside the tracks that the trains run on – this is mainly on the Underground lines, and some overground lines in London). The other uses overhead electrified wires, which power the train from above. These overhead wires are so powerful (25,000 volts) that the child doesn't have to touch them to be electrocuted – she just has to be near them. So if, for instance, a child dangles something over a bridge near these wires which enters their magnetic field, she will be in great danger.

Small children may climb through holes in fences, possibly vandalised by older children and which they normally wouldn't be able to get through, which will lead them to the track. British Railways Board ask you to report *immediately* any holes you see in these fences (to them or to the police) so that they can be repaired and your children can be protected.

British Railways Board produce an excellent, free booklet for children of five to ten years, to be read with parents – or on their own – called 'Roald Dahl's Guide to Railway Safety' (see below). It tells (or reminds) children about all the things they have to think about when playing *anywhere* near railway lines.

If any of these accidents happens, the child will be badly injured and will almost certainly have stopped breathing but may not still be 'live', that is, the high-voltage electricity may already have left the body – but you won't know.

This is a most terrible dilemma for any parent and most parents in this situation would be hard-pressed not to try and save their child's life. That is why I have pushed the Electricity Board Safety Department to tell me exactly when you can give first aid in this type of situation. (Their standard response is, 'You really shouldn't BUT you *might* be able to.')

LIGHTNING

If a child is struck by lightning, it has exactly the same effect on her body as a high-voltage electric shock EXCEPT that you can begin resuscitating her immediately without being electrocuted yourself.

The only thing you must be aware of is that in spite of the saying that 'lightning never strikes in the same place twice', it can. It would be better, therefore, if you can move her to a safer place, if there is one nearby – maybe away from the trees or, if it is practical, roll her down the slope to the bottom. Lightning always strikes the *highest* place. If she is clutching anything metal in her hand that she might have been holding before, prise it free – metal conducts electricity easily.

● Be aware that the child may have serious internal injuries.

● Start your ABC Resuscitation Routine immediately.

> A for **AIRWAY** (is it clear?)
>
> B for **BREATHING** (is she breathing?)
>
> C for **CIRCULATION** (is her heart beating?)

● Try to get someone to call for the ambulance, by dialling 999.

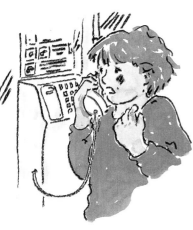

NEVER let your child go fishing in a thunder storm. *If lightning strikes it will be conducted through the carbon in the rod and your child could die.* Always remind children – and those going with them – that they must wind in their rods and stop fishing if there is a thunder storm.

If you would like the free booklet 'Roald Dahl's Guide to Railway Safety', you can get it from any large railway station or by writing to:

British Railways Board
Room 118, Euston House, 24 Eversholt Street, PO Box 100, London NW1 1DZ.

- Switch off the electricity OR move the child away from supply.
- DO NOT TOUCH THE CHILD *until you have knocked away appliance* with wood (brush handle) *dry* rubber (gloves) or paper (rolled-up newspapers, telephone book) OR turned off the supply.
- Treat her for shock. If the child is breathing, reassure and comfort her.
- If the child wants to be sick or is having trouble breathing, roll her over quickly into the Recovery Position.
- Dial 999 for an ambulance. Tell them what has happened.
- Treat any burns. REMEMBER *there may be burns* where the electricity entered and left the body, as well as bad internal burns.

THINK

- Have you got help? Try shouting out of the window or front door.
- Have you called the ambulance? Try to get someone to do this.
- Have you checked for DANGER?
- Shake and shout to the child to see if she is conscious.

IF THE CHILD IS UNCONSCIOUS: be ready to start your ABC RESUSCITATION ROUTINE.

Now check   'A' for AIRWAY – is it clear?

IF SHE DOESN'T RESPOND: OPEN THE AIRWAY. Tilt the child's head back and lift her chin forward. REMEMBER babies' necks are chubbier and more fragile. **Be gentle yet firm enough to tilt head back so airway is open.**

Now check   'B' for BREATHING

LOOK
LISTEN ⎬ for breathing
FEEL

IF THE CHILD IS NOT BREATHING: BREATHE FOR THE CHILD. Cover her mouth, or nose and mouth, with your mouth. Give her FIVE separate breaths. Watch her chest rise with each breath. *Less* breath for babies.

Now check   'C' for CIRCULATON

Is her heart beating? Check for the pulse. Feel the neck (or arm in a baby) for pulse. **If there is no pulse and you haven't got help GET IT NOW.**

IF YOU CANNOT FEEL A PULSE: DO CHEST COMPRESSION. Feel for the right place – one finger-breadth below the nipple line. Press on the chest, at a rate of **100 presses per minute.**

For children over one year old: Use the 'heel' of one hand only, with your arm straight. **Press fifteen times to every two breaths** (so your hand presses in about 2.5-3.5cm or 1-1½ inches each time).

For babies: Use two fingers only and **press five times to one breath** (so your fingers press in about 2cm or about ¾ of an inch, each time).

KEEP DOING THIS UNTIL THE AMBULANCE ARRIVES.

16 EYE INJURIES AND INFECTIONS

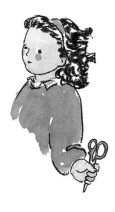

When a child hurts an eye, it is really important to know exactly what has caused the injury. Did something fly or blow into it? Did something splash into it, such as a chemical? Was it scratched by a branch of a tree or a sharp object? Or the eye may have been cut or bruised by a direct blow, or by falling onto glass (such as a child's glasses breaking as she falls over), or sometimes by school things being stuck in the eye. Hospital Accident and Emergency departments are constantly admitting children who have had eye accidents with pencils, compasses or scissors which they were holding when they fell over. Tell children never to run with scissors and sharp instruments in their hands. If they are walking around with them show them how to hold them safely.

Even if a child has not had an obvious injury, but you see her constantly rubbing a red, watery eye, or she complains that it hurts or itches, you must suspect an eye injury and take the situation seriously.

The eye tissue is delicate and unfortunately once any part of the eye is scarred the child's eyesight may be affected for the rest of her life.

WHAT TO LOOK FOR

If your child has something in her eye, this is what it will look and feel like:

● It will be painful, red and sore, or itchy.

● The eye will be watery.

● She may not be able to see out of it, although there may be no obvious injury.

● It may, of course, be bleeding.

The most usual things that children get in their eyes are bits of dust, sand or grit, or even loose eyelashes. If they are not dealt with quickly, they can cause scratches on the outside of the eyeball that are painful and which can cause scarring, infection, and damage to the child's sight.

There is a thin film covering the whole surface of the eye (the con-

146

junctiva). It is rather like a spider's web in so far as things stick to it and are difficult to get off once they are there. Unless you are careful you can cause more damage trying to remove anything that is stuck to it, rather than leaving it there and letting the hospital deal with it.

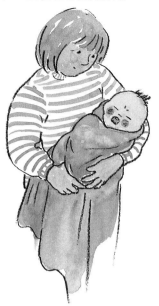

WHAT TO DO

If your child is a baby or toddler:

● Reassure and comfort the child. She will be in a lot of pain.

● You need to stop the child wriggling so that you can look in her eye. The simplest way to do this is to wrap the child up firmly in a blanket or sheet, so that her arms are inside and she can't rub her eye. If your child is calm and will allow you to look at and, if necessary, wash out her eye – without trying to stop you – then you don't have to hold her like this.

● Open her eye gently, using your index and middle fingers to separate the lids. Be careful if you have long or sharp nails.

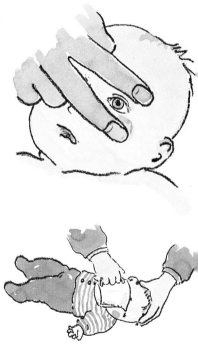

● If you can see clearly what is in the eye, lie the child on the floor and quickly wash it out with cold water. *You must tell her what you are going to do calmly and clearly before you start.* Use a feeding cup with a little spout, if you have one, or a jug. (It is worth buying a feeding cup and keeping it with your first aid kit. Or you may find an eye-wash bottle useful. You can get these at specialist chemists. You fill them with cool water and spray gently into the eye. The water will wash away any foreign body even more easily than if you use the feeding cup or jug.) Rinse the eye from the inner corner to the outer corner, tilting her head towards the side of the bad eye.

● If the object does not wash out immediately, cover her eye with a piece of clean gauze wrapped round a pad of cotton wool. Ideally, use a sterile eye-pad (see page 282, First Aid Kit). Tie the dressing lightly around the head with a bandage. If she struggles and you feel that by putting this pad on she is getting more distressed, then don't bother. *But you must not let her touch her eye.*

● DO NOT cover the eye if there is something sticking out of it.

● Take the child to your local hospital Accident and Emergency department. (It is always better to take eye injuries to hospital rather than your GP, because doctors may not keep the special equipment in their surgery that is needed to examine the eye.) It is important that the child is seen quickly by a doctor specialising in eye injuries and diseases.

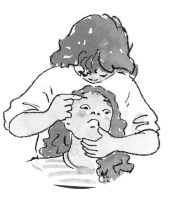

If your child is four years of age or over, and old enough to understand what is happening:

● Tell the child she must NOT rub her eye – she will want to, and it will be difficult for her not to.

● Ask her to sit down facing the light – preferably the window – and ask her to tilt her head back, as she might at the hairdresser's.

● Stand behind her and rest her head on your tummy.

● Reassure and comfort her that you are not going to touch the eye just yet, you just want to have a look. If the eye hurts a lot she may not want you to touch it. Try to persuade her to let you just have a look.

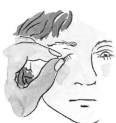

● Open up her eye using your index finger and middle finger to separate the lids. Be careful if you have long or sharp nails.

● Ask her to look left, right, and up and down.

● If you can see a little bit of dust, or an eyelash, under the top lid, gently pull the top eyelid over the bottom lid.

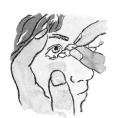

● If the speck of dust or the eyelash is either on the lower lid or is floating about the white part of the eye, wash your hands, and roll a damp corner of a clean tissue between your fingers, then gently see if you can lift it off the eye or lid. DON'T POKE if it doesn't come away from the eye almost immediately. If you can see clearly what it is, wash out the eye with water. Tell her what you are going to do before you begin.

● Using a feeding cup with a little spout or a jug, rinse the eye from the inner corner, towards the outer. Ask the child to lean her head towards the side of the bad eye.

● *If you can't get the object out of the eye right away, leave it* – DON'T FIDDLE. Just get her to hospital as quickly as possible.

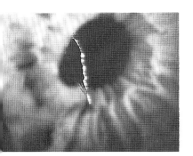

This is a scratch on a child's cornea. The scratch shows up after fluorescent drops are put into the eye. The doctor then looks in the eye with a special torch.

If having looked at the eye, and then having washed it out, you still cannot see anything but the child continues to complain *for longer than two hours*, you must take her to hospital. She may possibly have scratched the cornea and you cannot see this with the naked eye.

If the object is larger than just a speck, don't try to wash it out, just get the child straight to hospital. Cover her eye with a piece of clean gauze wrapped around a pad of cotton wool, or ideally a sterile eye-pad, and tie it lightly round the head. But if she doesn't want you to do this, leave it and get her to hospital.

If there is something sticking out of the eye, DON'T attempt to cover it, just get her to hospital as quickly as you can.

Never try to remove anything that is on the coloured part of the eye (the iris) or the inner dark circle (the pupil) (see Chapter 2 on How the Body Works), or try to remove anything that you think may be *stuck* in the eye. Just cover the eye with a clean, dry cloth if the child will let you (otherwise leave it) and get the child to hospital.

Never use a dirty handkerchief or cloth to cover the eye – this can lead to infection. *It is better not to cover the eye at all if you can't find something clean.*

CHEMICAL BURNS TO THE EYE

There are many corrosive chemicals – liquids, solids and powders – that can get into the hands and then the eyes of curious, unthinking or *unknowing* children, and they can cause tremendous damage, including blindness. They include many of the things that we use every day in the kitchen or around the house – oven cleaners, floor and wall cleaners, bleach, dish-washer powders and liquids.

WHAT TO LOOK FOR

If a child has splashed her eye with one of these chemicals, the eye will look and feel like this:

- She will have severe burning and itching in the eye.

- She will hold her eye tightly closed because letting the air and light in will make it hurt more.

- Her eye will be red, watering a lot and probably swollen – there may be burning of the skin around the eye.

WHAT TO DO

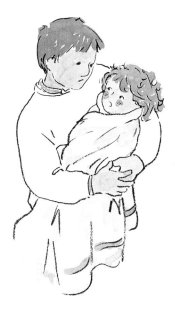

Whatever age the child is you must act quickly. *The quicker you can wash the chemicals away from the eye the less damage will be caused.*

- *Do not allow her to rub her eye.* If you have to – and I know it sounds harsh – hold her hands down, telling her what you are doing and why you are doing it. If the child is small enough you can wrap her up in a blanket with her hands inside to stop her touching the eye. Then, explaining what you are doing in as gentle a voice as you can, hold her under your arm, with your hand supporting her head.

- *Hold the injured eye under water poured gently from a jug,* holding her head to the side of that eye, so that the chemical doesn't spill over or splash into the good side. If her eye is very tightly shut in pain, you may have to prise it open gently, so that the water can get inside the eye. You MUST get water into the eye somehow. Be careful if you have long or sharp nails.

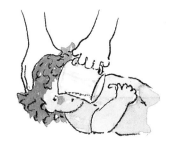

● REMEMBER, *you must get some water onto or into this eye*, so if you are not near a basin, or you are on your own and she is too big to lift to the sink – or too hysterical – lie her on the floor, with her head leaning towards the damaged eye, and gently pour water from a jug over the eye. Pour it from the inner corner to the outer corner of the eye. If you don't have water to hand, you can use milk, lemonade or beer, or anything bland, so that the chemical is washed away as much as possible *before you take her to hospital*. The quicker you wash the eye out, the less damage will be done.

● It is really important that you *tell her what you are going to do at each stage*. The pain of chemical injuries to the eye can cause severe shock and if you suddenly hold her head under cold water without telling her it could easily make things worse. This is particularly difficult with small children because they don't understand what is happening – you just have to cuddle them and be as gentle as you can.

● *Put a light dressing over the eye*, such as a piece of gauze over a pad of cotton wool, or a sterile eye-pad (see pages 281-283, First Aid Kit), and bandage it lightly in place. Alternatively, if the child struggles and really does not want the eye covered, leave it. As long as the eye is washed out, just *get her to hospital as quickly as you can*, making sure you keep her hands away from the eye.

● If you haven't done so already, dial 999 to call the ambulance. Alternatively, you may want to take her yourself by car to the hospital Accident and Emergency department or the Eye Hospital (if you have one near you).

EYE WOUNDS

WHAT TO LOOK FOR

If the child has grazed, cut or bruised her eye, for whatever reason, the eye may look and feel like this:

● She will almost certainly be in a lot of pain.

● The eye may be bloodshot or you may be able to see a wound on the eyelid or eyeball.

● The child may not be able to see out of the eye, or only be able to see out of it a little bit. There may be no obvious injury.

● There may be some clear fluid or blood (or both) coming from the eye wound. If this is happening – particularly if there is clear, straw-coloured liquid oozing out – the eyeball may look a funny shape and appear flatter than normal. This is because the fluid from behind the eyeball which gives it its rounded shape is oozing out. This is an extremely serious injury that needs *urgent medical attention*.

WHAT TO DO

- If you can, get someone to call for an ambulance. Tell them to say the child has an eye injury and to give as much information about the accident as possible.

- Reassure and comfort the child. She will be frightened and in a lot of pain. Hold her hand if you can. She can't see you but she can feel you and hear you, and these things will comfort and calm her.

- Lie her down on the floor (or ground, if you are outside) and support her head, to keep it as still as possible. If she is thrashing around with pain, tell her as gently and as calmly as you can how important it is to keep still. This is because if she cries, screams or coughs there is a danger that the pressure inside the eye could build up and she could lose fluid or more fluid from the eyeball which cannot be replaced.

- DO NOT try to remove anything which appears stuck in the eye.

- DO NOT try to put a dressing or cover on the eye. You will waste precious time.

- Treat the child for shock while you are waiting for the ambulance (see Chapter 27 on Shock).

REMEMBER – SHOCK LOOKS LIKE THIS

- Her face may be very pale and grey-looking
- Her skin may feel cold and clammy
- Her pulse may feel fast and weak
- She may be frightened and fidgety
- She may be very thirsty
- She may yawn and 'gasp' for air
- She may say everything feels fuzzy
- She may become unconscious

There are three important DO NOTs to remember when treating any eye injury:

1 DO NOT delay. If you are worried about your child's eye in any way, take her to hospital. It is always better to be safe than sorry when it comes to eyes – if you get it wrong and don't see a doctor, you cannot undo the damage that may have been done.

2 DO NOT give anything to drink in case she has to have a general anaesthetic.

151

3 DO NOT get anything from the chemist without your doctor having seen the child. Eye-drops and ointments may 'mask' the symptoms – that is, they may take the pain away, but in fact the eye continues to get worse.

EYE INFECTIONS

You might think that your child has an eye infection if her eye is watery, red and itchy. You might be able to see some yellowy discharge (pus), particularly if you press gently but firmly *with a clean finger*, underneath the inner corner of her eye. One clue is if the eyes are stuck together in the morning when she wakes up. This is most unpleasant and some children will be really frightened.

WHAT TO DO

- Rinse the eye with cooled boiled water which has a pinch of salt added to it – make it up in a clean jug or bowl. Support the child's head in the 'hairdresser's' position and (with very clean hands) soak a piece of cotton wool in the salty water. Gently wipe the eye from the *inside corner of the eye to the outside* – throw this piece of cotton wool away. Do this until the child can open her eye again or until most of the pus has been washed away. (This yellow pus is highly infectious, so you have to wash your hands after doing this.)

- Take the child to the doctor as soon as you can. He will give you some ointment or drops to put in the child's eye. As with antibiotics, you must continue the treatment for as long as it says on the box.

- Tell the child not to rub her eye.
- Reassure and comfort the child.
- Tell her what you are going to do.
- Treat her for shock.
- Wash out the eye with water, DON'T fiddle. If the object doesn't wash out immediately, get the child to hospital.
- Put a clean cover over the eye. If an object is sticking out of the eye, DO NOT remove it, DO NOT cover it. Just stop the child from rubbing or touching the eye – wrap her up in a blanket with her arms tucked inside.
- Call the ambulance by dialling 999. Tell them what has happened.

CHEMICAL BURNS

- *Splash the eye quickly with water or milk.*
- DO NOT allow the child to rub or touch her eye. Wrap her up gently but firmly, so that her hands can't reach the eye.
- Treat her for shock. The pain of chemical injuries to the eye may be bad enough to cause severe shock.
- If child wants to be sick or is having trouble breathing, roll her quickly into the Recovery Position.

THINK

- Have you managed to get some help? Try shouting out of the window or front door.
- Have you called the ambulance? Try to get someone to do this for you.

17 FITS

A fit (seizure or convulsion) is caused by 'a temporary electrical storm' in the brain causing some of the nerve cells to produce excess electrical activity. This means basically that the brain goes into overdrive.

Children can usually deal with this 'overdrive' without any obvious disturbance. The brain is able to recognise a danger point, and manages to defuse it automatically.

Some children, however, cannot deal with it; the brain becomes confused and loses control and they have a fit.

Four out of every hundred children will have a fit of some sort before they are five years old. The fit may be caused by a variety of reasons including epilepsy (see below); injuring their head and possibly fracturing their skull (see Chapter 19 on Head Injuries); meningitis (see Chapter 20 on Headaches); and high temperature.

EPILEPSY

There are three main sorts of epileptic fit: generalised tonic clonic; generalised absence; and partial fits. The British Epilepsy Association prefers these terms to others such as 'major' and 'minor' fits, which they feel can give the wrong impression.

Generalised tonic clonic

This type of fit is so called because it affects the whole of the brain; it may also be called Grand-Mal. In this sort, the child seldom gets a warning that she is about to have a fit; although rarely she will get a funny taste or be aware of a peculiar smell beforehand. Her body stiffens, often with a cry – this is not a cry of pain, it is just all her muscles going into spasm including the larynx (voice box) which forces the sound out.

She will fall to the ground and have a convulsion. She will thrash around and may froth at the mouth. She will almost certainly be blue in the face (because of lack of oxygen) and may wet or soil herself. It is this that causes children the most anxiety, particularly teenagers.

This episode may last only a few minutes during which she will be unconscious and unaware of her surroundings. She will then probably sleep, sometimes for a few hours, sometimes a lot less. However, it is really important to let her sleep for *as long as she wants to*, otherwise, if she is disturbed, she might fit again.

Generalised absence

This used to be called Petit-Mal (it is still by many doctors) and also affects the whole brain. In this type of fit the child does not fall to the ground because the muscles are not involved. She just doesn't see you. She will stare blankly ahead or she may blink or twitch slightly. These episodes last only a few seconds, and if parents are not looking out for them they may not notice anything unusual.

Even though she is standing (or sitting) the child will lose consciousness, but only for a second or two. She won't lose control of her limbs or become incontinent (in other words she won't wet or soil herself).

The danger for a child with this sort of epilepsy is that she will stop whatever she is doing at the moment of the fit. So if she is riding her bicycle she will fall off; if she is crossing the road she'll stop. Less important, but disruptive in its own way, is that if she is sitting in lessons at school she may just 'switch off'.

(This does not mean that all children who find it difficult to concentrate at school have epilepsy. She may just be bored or may have needs of a different kind that may not be being attended to.)

This condition is rare and a teacher may never have come across it before. It is hardly surprising therefore that children who have 'turns' can be thought to be 'lacking in concentration', 'disruptive' (when they try to find out from classmates what they have missed) and so on. It is really important that there is good communication between parents and teachers to prevent misunderstandings.

It is also important that parents understand what is involved in this sort of epilepsy. The diagnosis by the doctors is based almost entirely on what the parents tell them has been happening. Watch your child closely and paint as accurate a picture as possible.

The 'absence' episodes can be as upsetting and disorientating for a child as the fall-to-the-ground type of epilepsy.

Partial fits

These affect only part of the brain. They are divided into 'complex' and 'simple'.

The complex ones may start with an 'aura' or warning. This may be a funny taste in the mouth, some flashing lights, or a peculiar sound that the child hears.

There is no fit as such but the child may not appear to know you are there, and won't respond to you in the usual way. She has no control over what she is doing and may start to do odd things like plucking at her clothing or smacking her lips. She may also wander into dangerous situations while she is in this state.

In 'simple' fits the child may just have a funny feeling or jerk some part of her body, but not all the muscles are involved and she remains conscious. She is, however, 'out of contact' during this time.

Some children have a mixture of different types of fit, which is sometimes more difficult to treat.

Brain disturbance causing fits may also happen in other situations including:

- Diseases affecting the brain, such as meningitis.

- Severe head injury, such as a depressed skull fracture.

- Brain tumour.

- Diabetes.

- An overdose of (or severe reaction to) some drugs.

It is important for parents and carers to understand that although it is very unusual for a child to injure herself during a fit, it may be that if she fits a lot, or the fits themselves run into one another, she could become brain damaged. Doctors need to understand *why* a child is fitting and they may want to do a lot of tests on your child to see if she has a disease that is causing her to fit.

Children who have epilepsy want to be treated like children who haven't. So don't molly-coddle them. Having said that, it is important to recognise the first signs that need medical diagnosis and treatment. Once a child is 'stabilised' on treatment (in other words, once she has the right drugs to control the fits) she really can, and *should*, lead a normal life.

But what do you do for the first fit or the one that takes you by surprise?

It is important to remember that you cannot stop an epileptic fit, neither can you shorten its length. Once the child has the first sign (whatever it is) the fit will take on a life of its own.

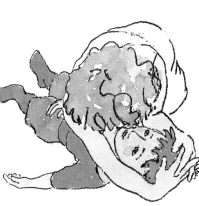

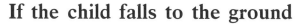

WHAT TO DO

If the child falls to the ground

- Move away any hard objects that she might strike herself on while she is thrashing about on the floor.

- Cushion her head with your hands or forearms, but don't try to prevent any movements. Go with her movements, trying to protect her as much as possible.

- DON'T put anything between her teeth. This used to be done, but is now considered dangerous – she could bite and break what you have given her and inhale the broken bit. Alternatively, she could break her teeth.

- DON'T try to move the child during the fit unless she is a danger to herself or to other people.

- As soon as the fit is over, roll her gently into the Recovery Position. Make sure her airway is open and that she is breathing easily.

- She may wet or soil herself and may be more distressed about this than anything else when she comes round. Tell her it is all right and try not to make too much fuss. Tell her what you are going to do; and clean up as best you can. If she is an older child, do the minimum necessary and then let her clean herself, if that is what she would prefer. (Perhaps this is something for you and your child to discuss at some point. She can tell you what she would rather you do in these situations. It is important that she knows that she is not alone and that you are trying to help her tackle this difficult problem together.)

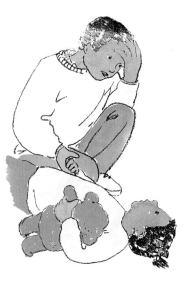

- Comfort and soothe her. She may drift in and out of sleep at this stage and won't be feeling well, but hearing your voice will calm her. Cuddle her if she wants you to, but otherwise find her favourite teddy or toy – anything that is familiar and loved will help – until she is feeling better.

- Stay with her or near her until she is fully recovered, but don't stimulate her too much. If you feel like playing a quiet game with her or reading her a story that's all right, but if she comes around too quickly there is a danger that she might fit again.

You only need to send for an ambulance:

- If it is a FIRST fit and you don't know why it has happened.

- If she has had a head injury and is 'fitting' soon after the accident.

- If during a fit she has injured herself and the injury needs urgent medical attention such as stitches.

- If the child has a second or third fit without coming round in between, in other words if she has one continuous fit.

- If the fit lasts more than two or three minutes LONGER than fits she has had in the past.

If the child has an 'absence' or 'complex' fit

In other words, if the child does not fall to the ground:

- Comfort and soothe her. Hearing your voice will calm her and there is no doubt that the calmer she is during these 'turns' the less traumatic they will be.

- Move any hard or dangerous objects on which she could hurt herself.

- Guide her away from danger spots such as the fireplace. Explain to her what you are doing and why you are doing it, whether or not you think she can hear you.

157

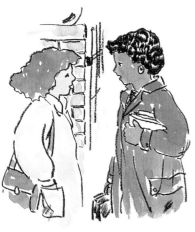

For a child who has any sort of epileptic fit it is important to tell child-minders, friends' parents and school teachers as well as the family. The way you put this over is important, both for you and for the child, so that she doesn't feel ashamed and you feel you have said what you wanted clearly enough to be understood.

Children who fit often feel guilty and need to be reassured that there are thousands of others like them who have fits and lead normal lives. They also need to be reassured that they are not to blame.

A child with epilepsy will tell you that the worst that can happen to her is to have a fit when she is with people she doesn't know; especially those she wants to impress. On occasions, however, this may happen.

Children with epilepsy need to carry their own ID card to explain to anyone who finds them having a fit that they have epilepsy.

When I was a staff nurse in an Accident and Emergency department in London, we used to see children with epilepsy being brought in time after time. When they woke up they were often very upset to find themselves yet again in hospital, when what they really wanted was to carry on with their normal day.

This is a difficult situation for a first aider not knowing what to do for the best, and it is understandable that they dial 999 to be on the safe side. But from the child's point of view, people wanting to help should look first for the ID card and wait until the child comes round, and then ASK her if she wants to go to hospital. The answer will usually be NO (thank you) unless, of course, she has been injured during the fit and those injuries seem to need medical attention.

REMEMBER *the only time a child really needs to be in hospital* urgently is if she doesn't come out of her fit or one fit leads into another. This is a dangerous situation for the child. Call for an ambulance by dialling 999 and tell them what has happened.

If an ambulance has been called and if there is a Paramedic on board, he may give her the drugs she needs to stop her fitting, probably in the form of a suppository (this is given into her anus – back-passage). A member of the ambulance crew may also give the child oxygen to breathe in through a mask.

Once in hospital, depending on her condition when she arrives, the doctors will give her more drugs to control the fitting. They will also do all the investigations to find out why the treatment didn't work this time – if she is already taking anti-epilepsy drugs – or what caused her to fit, if it is the first time she has done this.

The British Epilepsy Association will provide up to five ID cards (so children can put one in every pocket and in their rucksack or satchel). They are free on request, once they have the child's personal details. Alternatively, once she is a member of the organisation, they will send her a posher credit card version. The cost of joining, at the time of writing, is £6.

The British Epilepsy Association is an organisation with lots of bril-

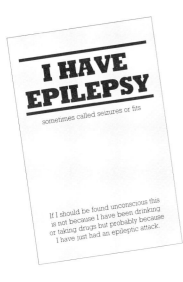

I HAVE EPILEPSY
sometimes called seizures or fits

If I should be found unconscious this is not because I have been drinking or taking drugs but probably because I have just had an epileptic attack.

liant ideas dedicated to helping children and parents to understand and cope with epilepsy. They have a range of excellent videos for hire and books and leaflets on all aspects of having epilepsy. They also have an *Adventure Club* which helps children to understand what epilepsy is about and more importantly passes on the message that plenty of children have epilepsy and cope with it. Contact:

The British Epilepsy Association
Anstey House, 40 Hanover Square, Leeds LS3 1BE.
Tel. 0532 439393.

Alternatively, you can telephone for help and advice for the cost of a local call on:

Epilepsy Helpline 0345 089599 Monday to Thursday 9 a.m. to 4.30 p.m., Friday 9 a.m. to 4 p.m.

FEBRILE CONVULSIONS

Febrile convulsions are fits due to high temperature. The unfortunate thing is that you can't tell which child, if any, will fit. For example, one child may cope very well with a thermometer reading of 40°C (105°F), whereas another will start to convulse (have a fit).

If you have a child who has these sorts of fits, I can only comfort you by saying that by the age of five she will probably have grown out of it.

Any infection of the nose, throat or ears can cause the child to have a high temperature and therefore to fit. A child with a high fever looks flushed and has an abnormally bright-eyed look. She may also be sweating.

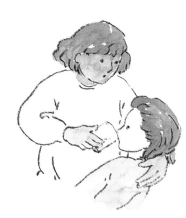

WHAT TO DO

The main thing is to try to prevent the fit from happening, BUT YOU HAVE TO BE QUICK. If the child has fitted before with a high temperature you will be more prepared (see 'Fever' in Chapter 22 on Minor Injuries and Illnesses); but *always try to bring down any high temperature as quickly as you can.*

- Once the temperature is up, give the correct dose of a paracetamol-syrup. The dose for your child's age-group is written clearly on the bottle or box. Every medicine is different so READ THE INSTRUCTIONS carefully.

- Give her plenty to drink. This will help to bring the temperature down. Encourage her by giving her something she really likes, perhaps in her favourite cup. This is better if it is not fizzy – it might make her feel sick – but if this is what she's used to and wants, let her have it. *The main thing is to get her to drink as much as possible.*

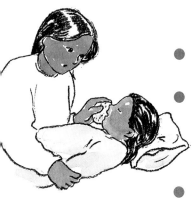

● If possible run a tepid (not warm, not cold) bath and sit the child in it. Get in as well if it is the only way that she will get in! Your aim is to get her temperature down, so although the child might say the water is too cold, you must gently persuade her to get in and have a splash about, as it will help to make her feel better. (She may not believe this at the time.)

● Do not in any circumstances leave her alone in the bath – *not even for a moment*.

● If you still can't get the temperature down, take the child out of the bath and damp-dry her. Don't dry her completely. Alternatively, sponge her down with tepid water making sure she or you sponges under her arms, behind her neck (particularly if she has long hair) and the backs of her knees.

● If you have an electric fan put it in her bedroom, NOT IN THE BATHROOM. (Or a fan heater may be used on cold.) Lie the child on her bed without any clothes or covers and put the fan near her – but not near enough to cause her any danger. *Tell her not to touch it.*

　　If you have no fan, open the window – but if the child is lying immediately beneath it, first move her bed from this position, or move the mattress. She won't catch cold and you must do everything you can to get this temperature down.

● Continue giving her drinks, even if she only takes sips – unless the child is being sick or cannot face drinking. If this happens encourage her to take small sips of cold water whenever she can.

● If the child starts to fit, DON'T GIVE ANYTHING TO DRINK. She could choke.

● Try not to cuddle her as this would increase her body temperature. Give her her favourite teddy or toy instead. In any case, feeling as poorly as this, she probably wants to be left alone. But she needs to know that you are around when she wants you.

● REMEMBER a high temperature often makes your child think horrid, frightening thoughts. You need to be there to reassure and comfort her and to explain to her what you are doing and why you are doing it. Don't just assume because a child is quiet that she isn't worried or frightened. She needs to hear your voice to be reassured that everything is all right.

● Keep taking her temperature. When it starts to come down you can close the window (or turn off the fan) and cover her *only* with a light sheet, cotton if possible. Do not let her wear pyjamas or a nightgown until her temperature has been below 40°C (100°F) for twelve hours.

　　It might comfort you to know that recent research shows that if you can prevent the child fitting in the first twenty-four hours of an illness, taking all the measures that I have described, it is less likely that the child will fit however high her temperature rises.

If the child starts to fit

WHAT TO LOOK FOR

- The muscles start to twitch and the arms and legs make odd jerking movements.

- Her eyes may roll backwards into her head.

- There may be some stiffness or arching of the back as the head is pushed backwards. Alternatively, she may just thrash her arms and legs about.

- She may hold her breath.

- She may go blue and the veins in her face and neck may stand out.

- She may froth at the mouth.

WHAT TO DO

Once a fit has started there is nothing you can do to stop it. It has a life of its own. So although it is a bit scary to watch, at this stage you can only keep her safe and STAY WITH HER.

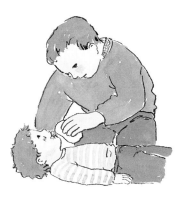

- Don't try to stop her thrashing movements but you can lie with her and 'go with' her movements to prevent her injuring herself.

- Remove any hard objects from the area to stop her hurting herself.

- Loosen any tight clothing, especially around her neck and chest.

- If she starts to 'bubble-up', in other words to produce so much froth from her mouth that she is in danger of inhaling it, wipe it away with a towel or tissue.

- If she is in the bath, take her out immediately.

Febrile convulsions should not last more than two, or at the most three, minutes. The longer the child fits, the more urgently she needs to be seen by a doctor. In some cases the doctor will decide that the fit must be stopped by a special drug called an anti-convulsant. This can be given by intravenous injection by the doctor. It may also be given in a small, lozenge-shaped suppository, by the Paramedic on board an ambulance.

   If the child fits for a long time there is a chance that she could stop breathing. This is very rare, but be prepared to carry out your ABC Resuscitation Routine.

161

> **A** for **AIRWAY**   (is it clear?)
>
> **B** for **BREATHING**   (is she breathing?)
>
> **C** for **CIRCULATION**   (is her heart beating?)

Once the fit is over

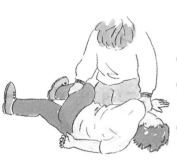

- Make sure she has plenty of fresh air – open the window or carry her to the front door. This is to improve her supply of oxygen and it may also help to cool her down. BUT wait until the fit is over – *a gulp of fresh air might start another fit*.

- Remove some of her clothes to help her cool down quickly.

- When she is breathing normally, roll her gently into the Recovery Position.

- Call the doctor, if this hasn't already been done.

NEVER LEAVE A CHILD ALONE WHO IS HAVING A FIT.

- Once a fit starts DO NOT try to stop it or try to move the child.
- Loosen any tight clothing around the neck and chest.
- Protect the child from injury by cushioning her head in your hands. Remove any hard objects from around her.
- DON'T put anything between the child's teeth.
- Once the fit is over roll her into the Recovery Position.

THINK

- Have you got help? Try shouting out of the window or front door.
- Have you called the ambulance? Try to get someone to do this.
- Have you checked for DANGER?

EPILEPTIC FIT – ONLY call for an ambulance if this is the child's first fit OR she has injured herself during the fit.

FIT DUE TO HIGH TEMPERATURE – If a child fits for a long time, she might stop breathing. Sponge her with tepid water (not cold, not hot) as soon as you can, to cool the child and stop her from fitting again.

IF THE CHILD BECOMES UNCONSCIOUS: be ready to start your ABC RESUSCITATION ROUTINE.

Now check   'A' for AIRWAY – is it clear?

IF SHE DOESN'T RESPOND: OPEN THE AIRWAY. Tilt the child's head back and lift her chin forward. REMEMBER babies' necks are chubbier and more fragile. **Be gentle yet firm enough to tilt head back so airway is open.**

Now check   'B' for BREATHING

LOOK
LISTEN } for breathing
FEEL

IF THE CHILD IS NOT BREATHING: BREATHE FOR THE CHILD. Cover her mouth, or nose and mouth, with your mouth. Give her FIVE separate breaths. Watch her chest rise with each breath. *Less* breath for babies.

Now check   'C' for CIRCULATION

Is her heart beating? Feel the neck (or arm in a baby) for a pulse.

IF YOU CANNOT FEEL A PULSE: DO CHEST COMPRESSION. Feel for the right place – one finger-breadth below the nipple line. Press on the chest, at a rate of **100 presses per minute**.

For children over one year old: Use the 'heel' of one hand only, with your arm straight. **Press fifteen times to every two breaths** (so your hand presses in about 2.5-3.5cm or 1-1½ inches each time).

For babies: Use two fingers only and **press five times to one breath** (so your fingers press in about 2cm or about ¾ of an inch, each time).

KEEP DOING THIS UNTIL THE AMBULANCE ARRIVES.

18 FRACTURES AND BONE INJURIES

Bones are a bit like the branches of trees when they are banged, twisted or strained. Old bones, like old branches, snap more easily than young, supple ones, which tend to split, bend or crack if given a heavy knock – like a young sapling.

Children, especially very young children, tend to crack their bones like this. It is still a fracture, but instead of breaking into two parts it splits and then stays in place after the injury. This is called a 'greenstick' fracture. In a very violent injury, however, children's bones will break in the same way as an adult's.

Basically the bones are there to keep the body shape but also to protect what is inside. So the skull protects the brain, the ribcage the heart and lungs, and so on. The nerves pass messages from the brain telling us when to move. They also carry messages from the bones, skin and other organs telling us when we have hurt ourselves (see Chapter 2 on How the Body Works).

A child's bones don't stop growing until he is between fourteen and fifteen years of age, but this does vary enormously from child to child (girls tend to mature more quickly than boys).

WHAT IS A FRACTURE?

Often parents say, 'It's not broken, only fractured', but they are the same thing. Doctors often write it on case notes in shorthand, like this #.

A fracture can be caused by a blow ON or NEAR the bone, which then causes the bone to twist or break.

The important thing about fractures in children is to recognise that they have happened. This may sound pretty obvious but in fact many are difficult to spot, especially in a child who has been playing and has not bothered to mention that he has had a fall.

WHAT TO LOOK FOR

You may not notice anything unusual but there will be:

- *Loss of movement.* The child will simply not want to move the part that has been hurt. This is because there is a strong built-in mechanism in children to protect the area around the fracture. (Adults on the other hand feel they should try and move it, even though their bodies are telling them not to.)

● *Loss of power.* Even if he can move it the child will have no power in the limb. With a broken forearm, for instance, the child would be totally unable to hold anything in his hand.

● *Swelling.* There will almost certainly be swelling around the damaged bone where there may have been some bleeding around the fracture.

● *Deformity.* There will often be a rather odd look about the limb. It may not be lying straight or it may have a peculiar dent in the middle of it. It just won't look like it was before.

● *Pain.* If the child tells you his arm hurts, you are probably going to have a look at it at some point, no matter how busy you are. But often because of the way children's fractures are, they may not actually feel any pain.

● *Tenderness.* If there is no pain, there will definitely be some tenderness when the area is touched, especially if you put any kind of pressure on it. The only time this may be difficult to judge is with an ankle injury when trying to find out whether the ankle is broken, strained or sprained.

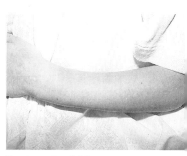

Fracture of a child's arm. This is what a limb looks like after it has been broken. Everything about it looks odd including its shape and position.

Only an X-ray in hospital will tell you accurately whether or not a bone is broken (see Chapter 2 on How the Body Works).

WHAT TO DO

Often after a bad fall the child may lose consciousness just for a moment and this is far more dangerous to the child than the fracture.

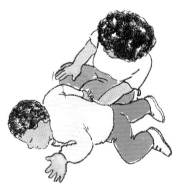

● He may be sick and his airway may block when you are least expecting it. If you have to leave him, for example to call for an ambulance, roll him gently into the Recovery Position. Try to do this without making him too uncomfortable. Ideally it is best not to leave him but get someone else to call for an ambulance.

ALWAYS roll him into the Recovery Position if you think he is feeling 'woozy' (saying the room is going round) or feels he is going to be sick.

● Treat the child for shock. Any child who has a bad accident, and sometimes even a minor accident, is likely to develop shock.

> ### REMEMBER – SHOCK LOOKS LIKE THIS
>
> - His face may be very pale and grey-looking
> - His skin may feel cold and clammy
> - His pulse may feel fast and weak
> - He may be frightened and fidgety
> - He may be very thirsty
> - He may yawn and 'gasp' for air
> - He may say everything feels fuzzy
> - He may become unconscious

- Try to prevent movement. A baby or toddler, having just fallen from the work-top for instance, may wriggle and scream not so much with pain but with the shock of having fallen from one level to another. The more you can prevent the child moving the injured bone, the less damage will be done to the nerves and blood supply and the less pain the child will feel. But with a struggling, frightened child this is easier said than done!

- Tell the child in quiet comforting tones what you think has happened and what you are going to do. Tell him you think he is going to have to see a doctor in hospital, but that you will be with him all the time. If you have other children and you have to make arrangements for them to be looked after, tell him that as well.

- To keep the injured part still you need to 'splint' it in some way by using something firm and solid alongside the now not-so-firm broken limb. This will support it and prevent it from moving as much as possible. The most immediate thing you will have near you is the child's own body. If you think he has broken a leg, tie it gently but firmly to the *other* leg.

Always make sure you tie above and below where you think the fracture might be, using long scarves (or large handkerchiefs on a small child) – anything to firmly hold and support the legs together. You must make sure that any joints, either above or below the injury – for example the knee and ankle joints in the case of a fracture of the lower leg – are padded and held firmly so that they cannot move. Any movement of the joint near a fracture will be almost as painful and do as much damage as the movement of the injured bone.

- If you think your child has broken his arm (wrist fractures are common in children when they put their hands out to save themselves from falling), use the child's own body again to support the injury. Bring up the bottom of his T-shirt or sweatshirt over his arm, tuck the arm into it, then pin it in place. Or gently bandage the bent arm to his chest, using a long scarf or bandage to support it and hold it in place.

- If the child has broken his fingers, gently bandage them together with those that aren't injured, telling him what you are doing and why. Then support his arm within his jumper, sweatshirt or anorak, making sure that the arm is kept as high as possible.

- If he has hurt his toes, then after bandaging them gently together raise his leg on cushions or pillows.

- *Always raise the limb* if you can do so without causing the child any more distress.

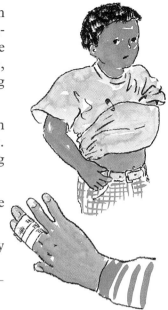

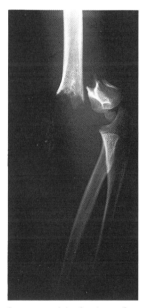

SUPRA-CONDYLAR FRACTURE

There is, however, one particularly bad fracture that children occasionally sustain which does need slightly more careful handling. This is a fracture of the inside of the elbow. It is called a supra-condylar fracture.

If you think your child may have a fracture like this, he certainly won't be able to bend his arm at all and will be in a lot of pain. If you can *you must stop the arm from wobbling about* as it is this that causes the pain.

You may not be able to support and 'splint' it because the arm may be sticking straight out in front of him or bent at a funny angle, and there is no way that he will let you touch it – *and neither should you try to*. The danger is that the bone may be pressing on the artery at the elbow. This child needs *urgent medical treatment* or he could lose the use of his arm.

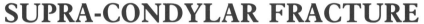

WHAT TO DO

- The best thing to do, if he is sensible or old enough, is to keep the fracture very still until the ambulance arrives. Ambulances carry special blow-up splints which are far less painful than anything you might try to put on him. However, he may be lying in too dangerous a place for you to leave him and you will have to protect this fracture before you move him. He may also be too young to understand what is happening to him and may be moving in pain and fear, making it worse every time he does so.

In this case, splint and support the arm with whatever you have to hand, making sure you keep it in the position that it is lying. Rolled up

Supra-condylar fracture of the elbow. This one is particularly nasty – as the lower end of the humerus (the long bone) in this child has been sheared off completely with the force of the accident. You can see how difficult it would be to splint it, or even keep it still!

167

magazines make a good splint – although you may have to tear them to make a smaller (child-size) roll. Alternatively, if you have any pieces of wood to hand they would be ideal. Then bandage these firmly in place, either side of the elbow.

Call the ambulance as soon as you possibly can by dialling 999.

If the child feels able to move, is not in too much pain and is not in shock, you might like to drive him to the hospital Accident and Emergency department yourself, *provided someone else goes with you in the car*. If he feels queasy or is sick, it is really important that there is another person there to look after him while you get on with the driving.

If you are not sure, wait for the ambulance.

The best thing for parents of a child with any type of fracture is to do *the least possible* to make him comfortable, and then get medical help as soon as you can. DO NOT give the child anything to eat or drink because he may have to have a general anaesthetic.

If your child becomes unconscious you must check his breathing and if it stops, start your ABC Resuscitation Routine.

> **A** for **AIRWAY** (is it clear?)
>
> **B** for **BREATHING** (is he breathing?)
>
> **C** for **CIRCULATION** (is his heart beating?)

When a child becomes unconscious one of two things can happen. The tongue can fall back in the child's throat and block the airway, or the child can be sick and within seconds can inhale it, blocking the airway in the same way.

There is a real risk that a child can die as a result of a fracture. This is not from the injury, but because the airway can become blocked and no one has *noticed*.

Once the child gets to hospital

He will have an X-ray and the doctor will be able to tell if he has or hasn't fractured the bone. Providing the fracture is not 'complicated' in any way – in other words the bone has not broken through the skin – the child may have a plaster of Paris cast. (This means the doctor, or technician, will put hard plaster-covered 'bandages' into a bowl of warm water to soften them, then gently bandage the child's injury over some soft gauze padding.) This then hardens quickly to provide solid support for the bones to heal. Some of these plaster casts are now made of fibre glass.

Very occasionally the child will have to go to the operating theatre first if the bones need to be pulled straight or if the broken bones have been pushed through the skin.

The child will usually be sent home from hospital after treatment. If it is a bad break or he has to go to the operating theatre he may have to stay in hospital overnight or at most for a few days.

As a general rule children with fractures of fingers, toes and noses are usually sent home; 'arms and legs' are usually kept in for observation; 'heads and backs' will always be kept in hospital until such time as the medical staff feel there is no chance of brain damage or paralysis resulting from the injury. But please remember every hospital is different (see 'Taking a Child to Hospital' in Chapter 1 on Preparation and Practical Issues).

19 HEAD INJURIES

Children fall on their heads rather a lot. Perhaps this is because, compared to adults, their heads are heavier and larger than the rest of their bodies and when they trip they tend to unbalance and topple over; or because they are just more adventurous. They also tend to get *hit* on the head much more than adults, probably because adults develop a sixth sense of danger which most children don't have.

Fortunately a lot of wounds to the head look worse than they are because they bleed a lot. This is because the scalp is well supplied with blood vessels and the skin over this area is tight, so that if it is knocked hard it tends to split open. If children don't bleed when they bang their heads, they tend to have very impressive, egg-shaped bumps.

The size of the bump or even the amount of blood may be alarming, and the bleeding may need urgent attention, but – more important – you need to know if her injury is severe enough to cause the child brain damage. You also need to think about whether she may have fractured her skull, although this is unusual in most head injuries to children. Fractured skulls are important to recognise but difficult to detect. There is a danger that if they are not picked up early enough the child may suffer from brain damage and might even die.

If you think that the child is not badly injured – she may only have tripped and bumped her head slightly – then lie her down for a while. If she has cut her head and any bleeding stops quickly, she is alert and *there is no drowsiness and no vomiting* there is probably no need to see a doctor.

BUT if you think she is behaving peculiarly, or if you are *unhappy about her condition in any way*, then you should get her to the doctor. If the accident happens in the evening, and you can't get to see your GP, take her to the hospital, or phone the ambulance by dialling 999.

WHAT TO LOOK FOR

REMEMBER there may be no bleeding after a head injury. In fact there may be very little to see.

● *She may be drowsy*. If she is old enough to talk she may slur her words or appear confused. Check on her at frequent intervals and if you are worried, wake her up in the middle of the night. This may sound crazy but if she really has given herself a serious bang you need to know that she is all right.

What you are trying to do by waking her is to see if she responds as

170

she normally would. Only you know your own child, but most children will talk to you if woken up and will be persuaded to take a drink and have a cuddle. If she is not her usual self – even if it is the middle of the night – and you are worried, you should call the doctor or take her to hospital.

- *She may complain of a constant headache* (if she is old enough to tell you). If she is younger she may pull her ears or may be irritable and obviously unhappy.

- *She may be sick.*

Any of these may require medical advice. The following signs will tell you that the child has been seriously injured:

- *There may be a soft 'boggy' area* on her head (with or without a wound nearby).

- *There may be blood or clear fluid leaking out of her ear or nose.* This is very serious and can result in permanent damage or disturbance to the brain, and in some cases a permanent handicap or death.

- *She may tell you that her eyes feel funny.* The 'images' she sees may seem blurred, or double, or she may not be able to see at all out of one or both eyes. If she is little she may sit and rub her eyes. This may or may not be serious, depending whether it is a sign by itself or whether there are other things that are making you worried.

  Her eyes may LOOK funny, or 'different' and when you look carefully at them you may see that her pupils are different sizes (see Chapter 2 on How the Body Works).

- *She may have a fit* (see Chapter 17 on Fits).

- The child may totally lose her memory (she may even be unable to tell you her name). With *any* loss of memory the child should always be checked out in hospital.

WHAT TO DO

Here are some guidelines to help you deal with your child's head injury, and to help you tell if it is a serious one:

- Lie the child down gently, reassuring her all the time. A child with a head injury might drift into unconsciousness. (Even when we bump our own heads it makes us feel peculiar for a few minutes.) If she can hear your voice and know you are there she is less likely to go into shock. Raise her head and shoulders slightly on a small cushion or folded-up blanket but make sure that her airway is not kinked, in case she loses consciousness and her breathing becomes difficult.

● If she looks as though she may be sick, roll her gently into the Recovery Position.

● Stop any bleeding, by direct pressure. To do this put a sterile dressing or clean fingers directly onto the wound. If there is something stuck in the cut in her head, put pressure *on the sides of it only*. (See Chapter 6 on Bleeding.)

● REMEMBER any child with a head injury might lose consciousness, so you must open her airway and check her breathing. If it stops, start your ABC Resuscitation Routine.

> **A** for **AIRWAY** (is it clear?)
>
> **B** for **BREATHING** (is she breathing?)
>
> **C** for **CIRCULATION** (is her heart beating?)

You must keep a close eye on her for the next twenty-four hours. Signs of brain damage, caused by these injuries, may have a slow beginning. Every child who has had any sort of bang on the head should be watched very carefully. It happens so quickly that it is often difficult to find out how serious it is at the time. If you have any doubts or if the bleeding does not stop seek medical help or advice.

When a child has an object stuck in a head wound

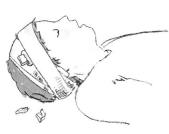

● NEVER remove any object – it may have gone into her brain and if you pull it out you could do even more damage or cause further bleeding.

● Cover the area around the sides of the object with a sterile or clean cloth. DON'T cover the object itself in case you dislodge it.

● Support the object on either side by building up the sides with padding. Bandage *around* the object.

If there is blood or clear fluid leaking from one of her ears

● Try to find something clean and soft to rest the ear against – such as a large pad of cotton wool, the inside of a large clean handkerchief or a wad of tissues.

● Bandage or just hold this lightly in place and then gently turn her over *onto the side which is leaking*.

● Be aware that she could become unconscious at any time. If she stops breathing, roll her gently over onto her back and start your ABC Resusciation Routine.

● Check her breathing rate and pulse at frequent intervals.

If she becomes unconscious, you need to know how deeply unconscious she is. You need to know your child's response to:

Sound (your voice)

Touch (shaking her gently)

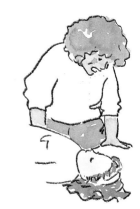

If there is some response, at either of these stages, the unconsciousness may only be light, but the danger is that she may sink into deeper unconsciousness very quickly.

If there is no response, then she is deeply unconscious and the brain activity is *dangerously depressed*.

If you haven't done so already, call an ambulance by dialling 999 and tell the Ambulance Service that the child has a head injury; give them as much information about the child's condition as possible.

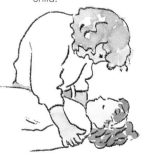

Shake and shout at the child.

Babies with a head injury

If a baby has a head injury or disease of the brain and the fontanelles – the soft spots on top of the head – are still open, she may behave very differently than an older child with the same injury (see Chapter 2 on How the Body Works).

WHAT TO LOOK FOR

● The fontanelles (soft spots) may bulge up and the skin over the area may feel tense and 'watery'. This may be due to bleeding inside the skull or a rise in pressure of the fluid surrounding the brain caused by injury or disease. Both are serious.

● The baby may be very irritable. Nothing you can do will soothe her and she may be anxious and restless. She will not want to feed or play.

● She may have a peculiar, high-pitched cry – very different from her normal one. This is due to pressure on the brain, either from 'brain fluid' or blood.

● She may thrust her head back in an odd sort of way, almost as if she is finding her head too heavy for her body. What this means is that her neck is becoming stiff and this is making her push it back in this way.

● The child may be sick a lot. (Being sick on its own is not a sign of head injury in a baby, but if it accompanies any of the other signs already mentioned, it is an important and serious sign.)

● She may have a fit (see Chapter 17 on Fits).

● She may become unconscious. In this case make sure she has a clear airway and check her breathing. Please remember babies have shorter

173

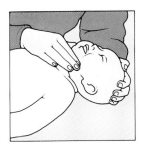

chubbier necks than older children and be aware of this when you are tilting her head back. Be prepared to start your ABC Resuscitation Routine.

A for **AIRWAY** (is it clear?)

B for **BREATHING** (is she breathing?)

C for **CIRCULATION** (is her heart beating?)

WHAT TO DO

- Do not wait for any further developments. The fluid pressure in the baby's brain is rising and the brain is getting squashed. If you don't act quickly, the brain cells will die and the child could have permanent brain damage. She may even die.

- This baby must GO TO HOSPITAL URGENTLY. Dial 999 to call for an ambulance and tell them that you think your baby has injured her head. Tell them what you have noticed the baby doing, so that they can be prepared for any emergency treatment to give her on her way to hospital.

WARNING
Hospitals are seeing an alarming increase in head injuries in children who are being shaken. *It is extremely dangerous to shake a child* because although you can't see any obvious injuries, it can cause internal brain haemorrhage and the child can become brain damaged or even die.

- Reassure and comfort the child.
- Lie her down. Tell her what you are going to do.
- If she wants to be sick or is having difficulty breathing, turn her carefully into the Recovery Position.
- If there is any blood or clear fluid leaking from one of her ears, roll her GENTLY *onto the same side as the injury*.
- Ring ambulance by dialling 999. Tell them what has happened.

THINK

- Have you managed to get some help? Try shouting out of the window or front door.
- Have you called the ambulance? Try to get someone to do this for you.
- Have you checked for DANGER?
- Shake and shout to the child to see if she is conscious.

IF THE CHILD BECOMES UNCONSCIOUS: be ready to start your ABC RESUSCITATION ROUTINE.

Now check   'A' for AIRWAY – is it clear?

IF SHE DOESN'T RESPOND: OPEN THE AIRWAY. Tilt the child's head back and lift her chin forward. REMEMBER babies' necks are chubbier and more fragile. **Be gentle yet firm enough to tilt head back so airway is open.**

Now check   'B' for BREATHING

LOOK
LISTEN ⎫ for breathing
FEEL ⎭

IF THE CHILD IS NOT BREATHING: BREATHE FOR THE CHILD. Cover her mouth, or nose and mouth, with your mouth. Give her FIVE separate breaths. Watch her chest rise with each breath. REMEMBER you need *less* breath for babies.

Now check   'C' for CIRCULATION

Is her heart beating? Check for the pulse. Feel the neck (or arm in a baby) for a pulse. **If there is no pulse and you haven't got help GET IT NOW.**

IF YOU CANNOT FEEL A PULSE: DO CHEST COMPRESSION. Feel for the right place – one finger-breadth below the nipple line. Press on the chest, at a rate of **100 presses per minute.**

For children over one year old: Use the 'heel' of one hand only, with your arm straight. **Press fifteen times to every two breaths** (so your hand presses in about 2.5-3.5cm or 1-1½ inches each time).

For babies: Use two fingers only and **press five times to one breath** (so your fingers press in about 2cm which is about ¾ of an inch, each time).

KEEP DOING THIS UNTIL THE AMBULANCE ARRIVES.

20 HEADACHES

Adults tend to think that children don't get headaches; but they do.

There are many different causes of headaches, most of which don't need first aid treatment other than a darkened room, perhaps a cold compress on the child's head, lots of comfort and reassurance, an occasional pain-killer such as paracetamol-syrup, and in some cases just food. If, however, the child is getting regular headaches or has a temperature, or if you are worried about her in any way, she should be seen by a doctor.

Children's headaches often go with a high temperature; small children with a temperature will probably complain of 'tummy ache', even though the 'ache' may be anywhere in their body.

COMMON CAUSES

Eye strain

If your child is short- or long-sighted and is straining to see the blackboard all day, she may develop headaches. If this happens get her eyes tested, but make sure the optician you go to is used to dealing with children.

Lack of food

Feeling hungry can cause headaches. Some children cannot cope unless they eat breakfast and have regular, non-sugary meals during the day. (Sugar will give the child an instant boost of energy but it won't satisfy hunger in the same way as a meal with protein and particularly carbohydrate – like bread or potatoes – will.)

Common cold

Colds, and possibly infection of the sinuses (sinusitis), can cause severe headaches and the child will need to be seen by the doctor.

Head injury

If the child has hurt her head or complains of headache, is unusually drowsy or is vomiting, she may have a head injury or a skull fracture. This child needs to be seen urgently by a doctor. (See Chapter 19 on Head Injuries.)

There are two other sorts of headaches which need attention, one more urgently than the other. They are meningitis and migraine.

MENINGITIS

Occasionally a headache is a sign of serious illness, particularly meningitis. This is caused by the lining of the brain (the meninges) becoming infected by a virus or bacteria.

Meningitis often attacks and affects the child so quickly that you may not have time to notice that the illness has become more serious than you first thought. It is no longer a matter of a child with a high temperature who needs lots of drinks, but a dangerously ill child who needs to be in hospital urgently.

This may be alarming for you even to think about but you must be AWARE and know how to recognise meningitis.

Remember, however, that most headaches are not meningitis.

Meningitis in children

WHAT TO LOOK FOR

- The child will be unwell with a recent ear or chest infection, and may already have seen a doctor.

- She is likely to have a high temperature, unless she is already being treated with antibiotics for another infection which may have brought any temperature down.

- She will complain of a severe headache, made worse by light and movement. It may be so bad that she will cry out in pain.

- She may be sick and become increasingly drowsy; she won't want to talk to you.

- She may tell you that her neck feels stiff; she may even thrust her neck back – this is a serious sign.

- She may be shivering.

- She may have hallucinations, not know who you are, and see people in the room who are not there.

- She may have a fit (see Chapter 17 on Fits).

WHAT TO DO

- If you feel there is even a possibility that your child is in the early stages of meningitis DON'T HESITATE to call the doctor. If the doctor is not available or it is the middle of the night then call for the ambulance immediately. Listen to what the doctor or emergency operator says and *do exactly as he or she tells you.*

177

Remember, doctors would rather answer a false alarm from parents than be called too late to be able to make the child better.

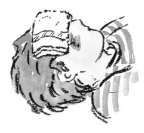

- DO NOT give any drugs (including paracetamol) unless they tell you to do so.

- This child will be frightened and will need a lot of comforting and reassurance.

- Darken the room by turning off the lights or drawing the curtains. Don't forget to tell her what you are doing. Stay with her.

- Ask her if she would like a cold compress on her head; this may help to relieve the pain.

- A bucket nearby may be useful in case she feels sick – these children may suddenly vomit.

- Hold her hand while it is really bad and tell her that she will be all right.

- Tell her the ambulance is on its way and that you are going with her to hospital.

- Remove any bedclothes or any easily removable clothes from her.

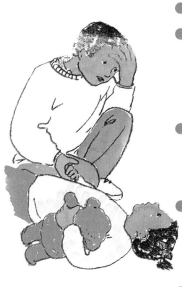

- Try not to cuddle her. It sounds terrible to advise you not to cuddle your own sick child, but holding her near to you will increase her body temperature. Instead give her her favourite teddy to hold. In any case if she is feeling as poorly as this, she will probably want to be left alone. But she will need to know that you are around when she wants you.

- REMEMBER having a high temperature often makes a child think horrid, frightening thoughts. You need to be around to reassure and comfort her and to explain to her what you are doing and why you are doing it.

- If you can, open a window or switch on an electric fan to cool her down.

WATCH HER CAREFULLY:

- While you are waiting for the ambulance watch for the difference between how the child WAS and how she is now. If she has meningitis, her condition may *get worse*.

- She could become drowsy, and may have a fit.

- If she is dangerously ill she will eventually become unconscious (see Chapter 31 on Unconsciousness). If you find your child in a state of unconsciousness you must open her airway and check her breathing; if it stops, start your ABC Resuscitation Routine.

A for **AIRWAY** (is it clear?)

B for **BREATHING** (is she breathing?)

C for **CIRCULATION** (is her heart beating?)

Meningitis in babies

Babies cannot tell you how they feel, so you have to be particularly watchful of a baby with a very high temperature.

WHAT TO LOOK FOR

The clues to look out for, apart from the temperature, are:

- Drowsiness and irritability. The baby may not want to be picked up, and she may raise her eyes up into her head in an exaggerated effort to try to get to sleep as soon as she is put in her cot.

- When she opens her eyes, she may seem 'vacant' and not be aware that you are there.

- She may have a peculiar, high-pitched cry that is totally unlike her normal cry. This is a very dangerous sign.

- She may develop some neck stiffness and arch her back, pushing her head back.

- She will probably refuse any feeds you give her but may be comforted by a suck on the breast. If she does take anything, however, she may be sick.

- Her fontanelles or 'soft spots' on the top of her head may bulge up rather than be level with the head, as they normally are.

- She may have a fit (see Chapter 17 on Fits).

- If she is dangerously ill she will become unconscious.

WHAT TO DO

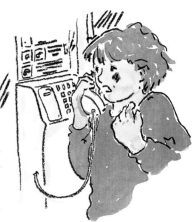

- You need medical help URGENTLY. Call your doctor or call for an ambulance by dialling 999. Tell them what has happened and do exactly as they tell you to do. DO NOT give any drugs – including paracetamol.

- Darken the room by turning off the lights or drawing the curtains. Stay with her. This will help to soothe a baby who is irritable and has a pain in her head.

179

- Try not to cuddle her too much as it will increase her body temperature. Give her a favourite toy or teddy instead. But don't forget she will be comforted by hearing your voice and knowing that you are near.

- Watch her carefully while you are waiting for the ambulance. The important thing to watch for is the difference between how the baby WAS and how she is now. If she has meningitis her condition WILL GET WORSE and she will become drowsy, and may have a fit (see Chapter 17 on Fits). She will eventually become unconscious (see Chapter 31 on Unconsciousness).

- If your baby becomes unconscious you must start your ABC Resuscitation Routine.

> A for **AIRWAY** (is it clear?)
>
> B for **BREATHING** (is she breathing?)
>
> C for **CIRCULATION** (is her heart beating?)

Once the child gets to hospital

Doctors and nurses will move quickly. Meningitis in children is a dangerous disease and they will want to do a lot of tests quickly.

One of the tests they will do is a lumbar puncture. This means putting a needle into the bottom of the child's spine and drawing off some fluid. (This is the fluid that 'bathes' the child's brain and spine, protecting them from damage and buffering from the outside world.)

She will be put on special antibiotics to fight the infection. The doctor will almost certainly put up a 'drip'. This means putting a needle into the child's vein and attaching it to a long tube which leads into a bottle. This literally drips vital fluid into her body to keep her from getting dehydrated.

The child may be kept in isolation, which may sound like a punishment, but it means that she will be nursed away from other children. The nurses will wear masks and gowns and you will be asked to do the same. She probably won't be allowed visitors other than you and your partner for the first few days – or until the infection is under control.

REMEMBER meningitis is highly infectious. If possible keep other children away, even if you only *think* the child has this infection. If your child or baby is diagnosed as having meningitis you may be asked for the names and addresses of the people she has mixed with in the last few days, so that they can be contacted and given antibiotics.

For further information contact the National Meningitis Trust, Fern House, Bath Road, Stroud, Glos, GL5 3JJ, Tel. 0453 751738 or, out of hours, 0453 755049.

There is now a national 'catch up' campaign to encourage parents to immunise all children under four years against HIB (Haemophilus influenzae type b) meningitis. You will receive a letter from your doctor inviting you to have your children immunised – starting with the youngest as they are most at risk.

MIGRAINE

Children are more likely to get migraine if they already suffer from an allergic illness such as asthma, eczema or hay fever. They are also more likely to get it if you had it as a child.

Migraines are horrible in so far as they 'take over' the child. There is nothing the child can do but give in to the pain, no matter how plucky she is. Some children go very pale, some are sick and some are both during a migraine attack.

A child with migraine should not be told to 'pull herself together' or 'not to be such a baby' when what she really needs is nurturing, reassuring and comforting.

If your child gets migraines from time to time, there are some things you should ask yourself:

- Does she tend to get these attacks after eating some foods? She may be allergic to them (see Chapter 4 on Allergies).

- Could her eyesight be the problem? Her eyes may need testing.

- Does she get these migraines when she is hungry or over-tired? Some early nights may help. (Don't expect her to agree to this.)

If you cannot think of anything that might trigger off the migraines and they are getting more severe or are coming more often, it is IMPORTANT that she is checked and assessed by a doctor.

WHAT TO DO

- She needs to be in a quiet, darkened room. She may see flashing lights and other horrible things and the darkness will help.

- A cold compress on her head will help to make her feel better.

- Paracetamol-syrup given in the right dose for your child, as written on the bottle, may help to take the pain away. (You may prefer a sugar-free sort if you can find one.)

- A bucket nearby will be useful if she feels sick; children may vomit suddenly.

- Hold her hand while it is very bad and tell her she is going to be all right. These attacks can be frightening, and fear makes them worse.

181

MENINGITIS (Read this section of the *chapter* carefully)

- Dial 999 for an ambulance. Tell them what you think is the matter.
- Try to cool the child down. If she is in too much pain to let you touch her, just take off the bed clothes or open the window.
- DO NOT give her anything to eat or drink.
- The child will be very frightened – reassure and comfort her.

IF SHE STARTS TO HAVE A FIT:

- Once the fit starts DO NOT try to stop it or move the child.
- Loosen any tight clothing round her neck and chest.
- Protect the child from injury. Cushion her head in your hands.
- DON'T put anything between her teeth.
- Once fit is over reassure and *roll her into the Recovery Position*.
- If the child fits for a long time, she might stop breathing.

THINK

- Have you got help? Try shouting out of the window or front door.
- Have you called the ambulance? Try to get someone to do this.

IF THE CHILD BECOMES UNCONSCIOUS: be ready to start your ABC RESUSCITATION ROUTINE.

Now check 'A' for AIRWAY – is it clear?

IF SHE DOESN'T RESPOND: OPEN THE AIRWAY. Tilt her head back and lift her chin forward. REMEMBER babies' necks are chubbier and more fragile.

Now check 'B' for BREATHING

LOOK
LISTEN } for breathing
FEEL

IF THE CHILD IS NOT BREATHING: BREATHE FOR THE CHILD. Cover her mouth, or nose and mouth, with your mouth. Give her FIVE separate breaths. Watch her chest rise with each breath (*less* breath for babies).

Now check 'C' for CIRCULATION

Is her heart beating? Feel the neck (or arm in a baby) for a pulse.

IF YOU CANNOT FEEL A PULSE: DO CHEST COMPRESSION. Feel for the right place – one finger-breadth below the nipple line. Press on the chest, at a rate of **100 presses per minute.**

For children over one year old: Use the 'heel' of one hand only, with your arm straight. **Press fifteen times to every two breaths** (so your hand presses in about 2.5-3.5cm or 1-1½ inches each time).

For babies: Use two fingers only and **press five times to one breath** (so your fingers press in about 2cm or about ¾ of an inch, each time).

KEEP DOING THIS UNTIL THE AMBULANCE ARRIVES.

Meningitis is very infectious. *Tell the medical team* if you resuscitated her.

HYPOTHERMIA AND HYPERTHERMIA

21

*Hypo*thermia means a *low body temperature*, where the child's body 'core' temperature has gone below a critical level and she is too COLD. (This is generally considered to be below 34°C or 95°F.) It is caused by the child not having enough clothes and protection from a cold atmosphere, whether it is inside or outside.

*Hyper*thermia means a *high body temperature*, where the child's body 'core' temperature has become overheated and she is too HOT. It can be caused from both *inside* the body – from an infection, for example, when the child has a temperature – and *outside* the body, if the child, usually a baby, is too warmly dressed or is put somewhere too hot, such as in the sun.

BABIES are most at risk from both these conditions. Most babies (and some children) have difficulty in regulating their own temperature. Therefore parents and others looking after them have to do it for them. This is sometimes difficult to get right.

In the first months of life babies can get cold very easily. The best way of keeping a baby warm is for her to wear a few layers of natural fabric (cotton or wool, if possible) including a vest, baby-gro or similar, and a cardigan. When she goes out she should always have a hat on when it's cold. Much of the heat from a baby's body is lost through her head – as it is with adults – so if she goes outside her head should be as snug and warm as her body. But remember to take it off once she gets inside, otherwise she will get too hot.

Once a baby is one month old she has a better chance of keeping herself warm, but she can't get herself cool again once she is too hot. At this stage she can wear the same amount of clothes indoors as an adult, as long as you keep her away from draughts. However, she will still have to be well wrapped up to go outside in winter. It is important to take the extra layers off, however, once she comes back inside.

Try to keep the house or flat at an even temperature. Don't worry about a baby getting cold at night – as long as she is wearing a nappy, vest and pyjamas or baby-gro and is tucked securely into her blankets, she will be fine. It is more important that she doesn't get too hot – you don't need to have the heating on if the room has been warm during the day.

DO NOT use a sheepskin (no matter how tempting the manufacturers make it sound) or a hot-water bottle for any baby. They are both dangerous in their own way (the sheepskin because the child could suffocate and the hot-water bottle because it could burn the child).

183

It may be difficult to know how many blankets to use on the cot, but *it will depend on what sort of blankets and how warm or cold the room is at night.*

This chart is a *guide* to how many blankets you might use.

Amount of bedding to use	Room temperature	
Sheet plus 4 layers of blankets	60°F	(15°C)
Sheet plus 3-4 layers of blankets	65°F	(18°C)
Sheet plus 2-3 layers of blankets	70°F	(21°C)
Sheet plus 1 layer of blanket	75°F	(24°C)
Sheet only	80°F	(27°C)

Duvets, baby nests and cot bumpers are not recommended for babies under a year old. They can cause suffocation (see Chapter 28 on Suffocation).

One way to tell whether your baby is warm enough is to feel her tummy – make sure your hands are warm before you do it though! Hands and feet may be cold but if her tummy is warm she is really all right.

If you want to be really sure that the baby is warm enough, you may want to buy a bedroom and nursery thermometer. This can be bought from:

The Foundation for the Study of Infant Deaths
35 Belgrave Square, London SW1X 8QB.
The price, at the time of writing, is £2.50.

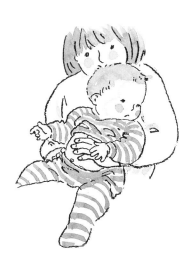

HYPOTHERMIA

Babies and very young children do not have the ability to shiver. Shivering is the way the body keeps the heat in and if the child's body is not mature enough to do this, her body temperature will drop more quickly.

Children generally, whether they are very young or not, do not cope too well in extremes of temperatures, particularly the cold.

WHAT TO LOOK FOR

This is what a child with hypothermia will look and feel like:

● A baby or child who is very cold may look extremely healthy because her face, hands and feet will be bright pink.

● Her behaviour, and how she feels when you *touch* her – particularly on her tummy – will give you the clue that all is not well.

● She may be quite grey-looking and her lips might look pale or blue.

● She will be unusually quiet, drowsy and limp. If she is little she will not cling on to you in her normal way but will just let go.

● She will show no signs of being interested in what is going on around her and she may even be confused – about you or where she is.

● She may be unconscious, or quickly become unconscious.

WHAT TO DO

This is a very serious situation and you must call for an ambulance immediately by dialling 999. The first thing you must check is that she is conscious. It is often difficult in cases of hypothermia to know whether a child is still breathing or her heart has stopped because everything slows almost to a standstill once the body gets really cold. There is a possibility that this child will have a cardiac arrest; in other words her heart will suddenly stop. You therefore have to watch her carefully and be prepared to start your ABC Resuscitation Routine immediately if you feel *fairly* sure that this has happened (see Chapter 3 on ABC Resuscitation Routine).

> A for **AIRWAY**   (is it clear?)
>
> B for **BREATHING**   (is she breathing?)
>
> C for **CIRCULATION**   (is her heart beating?)

● If she is breathing, put her in the Recovery Position, lying her on a coat or blanket until the ambulance arrives. Cover her with light layers of blankets or dry clothes.

● If she has been in extreme cold, such as on a mountainside or moor and especially if there is wind, rain, mist or snow, she is in danger of 'wind-chilling'.

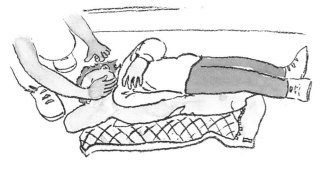
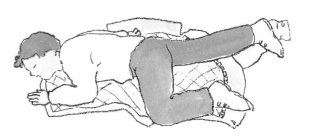

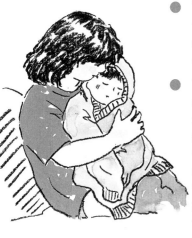

● Take off as many wet or damp layers as possible and replace them with warm, dry clothing. Then snuggle her inside your own clothes (if she is small enough) and carry her to a shelter. If you are going to lie her down, try if you can to put some layers *underneath* her.

● You need to get help quickly. If she is too big, or too badly injured to carry, or you are in a very deserted place and have no choice, you will need to take off some of your own clothes to cover her. Try to take off as much of her wet clothing as possible without moving her and then wrap her as best you can in your dry clothes. If you can't move her at all, just put your dry clothes over her wet ones. Remember to tell her what you are doing. Put her in the Recovery Position and go and call for medical help. Reassure her that help is coming and that you will try to be as quick as you can. However, if there is any other alternative, try not to leave her alone.

● If she can be carried inside, or was already inside when she got cold, she *must be warmed up slowly*. Do this by putting her on a material surface, such as on a blanket, a bed or even a carpet, and cover her with a few light blankets or layers of clothes.

● If you have any silver cooking foil to hand, wrap her in it and this will stop her losing any more body heat.

● If she is very cold and there is nothing else to hand, warm her with your own body by snuggling her inside your clothes.

● DO NOT use any direct heat like hot-water bottles or electric blankets.

● Keep reassuring her – she will be very frightened.

● If a child has been in a *near-drowning accident*, once you have done your ABC Resuscitation Routine take off any wet clothing carefully. If you can, towel her dry and put two or three *light* blankets, towels or clothes over the top of her. Don't be tempted to warm her up too quickly (see Chapter 13 on Drowning). You need to get medical help as quickly as you can. All children who have been in any kind of a near-drowning accident, *whether they have stopped breathing or not*, need to be seen in hospital.

● Do not give a child with hypothermia anything to eat or drink.

● Try if you can to get someone to call for an ambulance (see Chapter 1 on Preparation and Practical Issues). It is important that whoever is calling them gives very precise directions to the Ambulance Service, so that they can find you and the child quickly. Look around and try to find a landmark and describe it as best you can. Make sure you give the telephone number from where you are calling.

HYPERTHERMIA

The sweat glands in children, and especially in babies, are not well developed, so once they get too hot they cannot cool themselves down. If adults get too hot they sweat and this cools the temperature of the body. Once babies get hot, they just get hotter and hotter.

If the child is too hot INSIDE the body, in other words she has a temperature of 39°C (102°F) or over, you must cool her down.

The child will get too hot OUTSIDE the body either because she is too warmly dressed, or the room is too hot, or her pram or cot have not been protected from the heat – they may have been left in direct sunlight.

WHAT TO LOOK FOR

- Just be careful that if you have the heating on in the house or flat you always take a child's (particularly a little child's) outdoor clothes off quickly once you get inside – especially winter clothes, because they are so much more bulky.

- *A baby should never wear a hat indoors*, it will make her too hot.

- Never leave a baby sleeping either in the garden directly in the sun or by a very sunny window, where the glass *magnifies* the heat, making it even hotter.

- Never leave a child or baby in a car in direct sunlight. Apart from this being illegal, and the danger of them touching one of the car's controls, they will become hyperthermic in a very short time.

- Try to find areas for play that are shaded. Children burn in the sun very quickly (see Chapter 7 on Burns and Scalds).

- Never let babies or small children 'sunbathe' with or without sun protection cream. They should be kept well away from the sun by putting the hood of the pram up, by using a sun umbrella, or by putting the pram or push-chair in the shade.

- Be careful of wind-burn. It can cause as much distress as sunburn.

This is what a child with hyperthermia will look and feel like:

- In the early stages, the child will begin to feel unwell. She will feel dizzy and sick and may vomit.

- She will look flushed and hot (older children may look 'sweaty'). When you put your hand on her tummy it will feel hot and sticky.

- In the later stages of hyperthermia – if, for instance, she isn't dis-

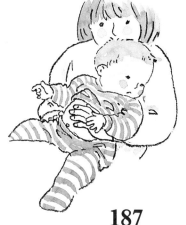

187

covered for a while – her skin will be hot and *dry*.

● She may be very restless, her breathing may be noisy and she may lapse into unconsciousness.

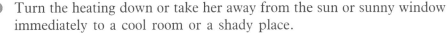

WHAT TO DO

This depends on what has happened and you will have to judge the situation according to the child's age.

If a baby or child has become over-heated from being over-dressed indoors or has been left in a sunny place, and although she is hot she is *alert* – in other words notices and responds to you – deal with it like this:

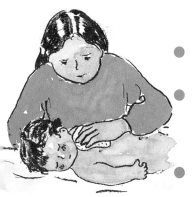

● Turn the heating down or take her away from the sun or sunny window immediately to a cool room or a shady place.

● Remove the blankets and covers from the cot or bed and, if her temperature is high, her clothes as well. If this doesn't work, you must sponge her down with tepid (not cold, not warm) water. *If a baby or a very young child is involved, and you are at all worried, call the doctor.*

● *She needs to have a lot of small drinks.* When babies and children are ill they often sleep a lot. However, if they sleep too long with a high temperature they can get dehydrated, in other words they lose too much fluid from their bodies. It is a good idea to wake the child up to give her a drink, but don't 'fill her up' with fluid in case it makes her sick. There is a slight chance that if her temperature continues to rise, *she might fit* (see Chapter 17 on Fits). If she begins to fit she will become unconscious and if she is sick there is a possibility she could inhale the vomit and block her airway. So although fluids are important they are much better in small sips.

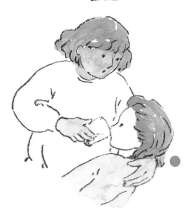

● *She may need medicine* such as paracetamol-syrup to help to bring her temperature down. The correct dose for your child is written clearly on the bottle. (You might like to try to use one which is sugar-free.) Never use an adult paracetamol preparation.

● NEVER give an overheated baby anything to eat.

However, if the baby or child is becoming drowsy – her breathing is noisy, and she is not alert (not aware of your being there) or she IS unconscious – DO NOT try to give her anything to drink. Treat her like this:

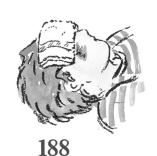

● You must cool the child as quickly as you can. Move her to a cool room or shady place and wrap her in a cold, wet sheet, or sponge her down with tepid (not warm, not cold) water, especially under her arms, in her groin and behind her neck, and put a tepid compress on her forehead. Leave the skin damp.

- Switch on an electric fan (or put on a fan heater on cold), and direct it towards the wet sheet or the child's damp body. Alternatively wave sheets, magazines, or anything else to hand, over her to try to get some draught to evaporate the water and to cool her body. This will help to reduce the temperature quickly.

- If the child becomes unconscious lie her down on a flat surface, open her airway, check her breathing and if breathing stops be prepared to start your ABC Resuscitation Routine. (See Chapter 3 on ABC Resuscitation Routine.)

> **A** for **AIRWAY** (is it clear?)
>
> **B** for **BREATHING** (is she breathing?)
>
> **C** for **CIRCULATION** (is her heart beating?)

- This is an emergency so get the child to hospital as quickly as possible, so that the dangerous amount of fluid that she will probably have lost from her body can be replaced. Ring for an ambulance, if you haven't already done so, by dialling 999. Tell them what has happened. (See Chapter 1 on Preparation and Practical Issues.)

- There is a possibility that this child could fit. Be aware of how to cope with it if she does (see Chapter 17 on Fits).

- In a child who has obviously over-heated, don't waste time taking her temperature. Just cool her down as best you can and wait for the ambulance.

SUNSTROKE

Remember that children can become over-heated out of the sun as well as directly beneath it. The danger times are:

- when it is sunny and windy and it is difficult to feel the heat;

- when she has been swimming and her body is wet;

- when a child is floating on the water on an air-bed or with water wings; the water reflects the sun, making it even hotter.

189

WHAT TO DO

If a child has sunburn on the parts of her body that have been exposed to the sun, such as her face, back or legs, and she is *not showing signs of being over-heated* (having hyperthermia), this is what you do:

- Move the child into the shade. Cool her by sponging her skin gently with cool/tepid water.

- If your child has been burnt by the sun, and the skin is swollen and blistered as well as hot, she needs to see a doctor urgently. (See Chapter 7 on Burns and Scalds.)

- Call the ambulance by dialling 999 and tell them what has happened.

- Reassure and comfort her (if her skin is burnt she may be in a lot of pain). She may also be in a state of shock (see Chapter 27 on Shock).

REMEMBER – SHOCK LOOKS LIKE THIS

- Her face may be very pale and grey-looking
- Her skin may feel cold and clammy
- Her pulse may feel fast and weak
- She may be frightened and fidgety
- She may be very thirsty
- She may yawn and 'gasp' for air
- She may say everything feels fuzzy
- She may become unconscious

- If she is alert (notices and responds to you) give her lots of *little* sips of cold water.

- If her breathing is noisy, and she is *not* alert (that is, not aware of your being there) do not give her anything to drink.

- If the child becomes unconscious you must open her airway and check her breathing. If it stops, start your ABC Resuscitation Routine.

A for **AIRWAY** (is it clear?)

B for **BREATHING** (is she breathing?)

C for **CIRCULATION** (is her heart beating?)

190

- Reassure and comfort the child.
- Get her to a warm place and snuggle her in your clothes. If she is too badly injured, too heavy or in too dangerous a place to do this, you may have to leave her to get help.
- If possible replace wet layers of clothing with warm layers instead (yours).
- Try to put layers of clothes underneath her, *as well as* on top.
- If you leave her: make sure she is in the Recovery Position and BREATHING.
- DO NOT give a child with hypothermia anything to eat or drink.
- DO NOT use direct heat (hot water bottle, etc.).
- Dial 999 for an ambulance. Tell them what has happened. *A child with hypothermia can sometimes become unconscious.*

THINK

- Have you got help? Try shouting out of the window or front door.
- Have you called the ambulance? Try to get someone to do this.
- Have you checked for DANGER?
- Shake and shout to the child to see if she is conscious.

IF THE CHILD IS UNCONSCIOUS: be ready to start your ABC RESUSCITATION ROUTINE.

Now check   'A' for AIRWAY – is it clear?

IF SHE DOESN'T RESPOND: OPEN THE AIRWAY. Tilt the child's head back and lift her chin forward. REMEMBER babies' necks are chubbier and more fragile. **Be gentle yet firm enough to tilt head back so airway is open.**

Now check   'B' for BREATHING

LOOK
LISTEN } for breathing
FEEL

IF THE CHILD IS NOT BREATHING: BREATHE FOR THE CHILD. Cover her mouth, or nose and mouth, with your mouth. Give her FIVE separate breaths. Watch her chest rise with each breath. *Less* breath for babies.

Now check   'C' for CIRCULATION

Is her heart beating? Check for the pulse. Feel the neck (or arm in a baby) for a pulse. **If there is no pulse and you haven't got help GET IT NOW.**

IF YOU CANNOT FEEL A PULSE: DO CHEST COMPRESSION. Feel for the right place – one finger-breadth below the nipple line. Press on the chest, at a rate of **100 presses per minute.**

For children over one year old: Use the 'heel' of one hand only, with your arm straight. **Press fifteen times to every two breaths** (so your hand presses in about 2.5-3.5cm or 1-1½ inches each time).

For babies: Use two fingers only and **press five times to one breath** (so your fingers press in about 2cm or about ¾ of an inch, each time).

KEEP DOING THIS UNTIL THE AMBULANCE ARRIVES.

- Reassure and comfort the child. Tell her what you are doing.
- You must cool the child's body down – but not too quickly.
- Move her away from the 'hot' place. Take any blankets or duvets off the cot/bed and take any clothes off the child.
- Cool the child by sponging with *tepid* water (not cold, not hot).
- Give lots of drinks *in sips*. DO NOT give anything to eat.
- Give paracetamol-syrup to bring temperature down.

If the child's body gets too hot there is a chance that she will fit. If the child fits for a long time, there is a small chance that *she might stop breathing*.

THINK

- Have you got help? Try shouting out of the window or front door.
- Have you called the ambulance? Try to get someone to do this for you.
- Have you checked for DANGER?
- Shake and shout to the child to see if she is conscious.

IF THE CHILD BECOMES UNCONSCIOUS: be ready to start your ABC RESUSCITATION ROUTINE.

Now check   'A' for AIRWAY – is it clear?

OPEN THE AIRWAY. Tilt the child's head back and lift her chin forward. REMEMBER babies' necks are chubbier and more fragile. **Be gentle yet firm enough to tilt head back so airway is open.**

Now check   'B' for BREATHING

LOOK
LISTEN } for breathing
FEEL

IF THE CHILD IS NOT BREATHING: BREATHE FOR THE CHILD. Cover her mouth, or nose and mouth, with your mouth. Give her FIVE separate breaths. Watch her chest rise with each breath. *Less* breath for babies.

Now check   'C' for CIRCULATION

Is her heart beating? Check for the pulse. Feel the neck (or arm in a baby) for a pulse. **If there is no pulse and you haven't got help GET IT NOW.**

IF YOU CANNOT FEEL A PULSE: DO CHEST COMPRESSION. Feel for the right place – one finger-breadth below the nipple line. Press on the chest, at a rate of **100 presses per minute.**

For children over one year old: Use the 'heel' of one hand only, with your arm straight. **Press fifteen times to every two breaths** (so your hand presses in about 2.5-3.5cm or 1-1½ inches each time).

For babies: Use two fingers only and **press five times to one breath** (so your fingers press in about 2cm or about ¾ of an inch, each time).

KEEP DOING THIS UNTIL THE AMBULANCE ARRIVES.

MINOR INJURIES AND ILLNESSES

22

This chapter is a guide to what you may want to do to help your child if he gets ill or injures himself.

If you are not sure what is the matter with him or what he has done to himself AND YOU ARE WORRIED, *you must not hesitate to call the doctor*, even if it is the middle of the night. Doctors would rather be called than not, even when it is a false alarm – especially when you have a young baby.

It is sometimes very difficult for parents to assess what is serious and what isn't.

BED WETTING

Some children seem to have to leave going to the toilet until it is (almost) too late. Others continue to wet the bed at night, especially if they are troubled. Try to understand if he has the occasional accident in this way. Be aware that a lot of boys (boys more than girls) continue bed wetting until five years of age, so don't worry too much – it's just a nuisance for you, and the less fuss you make, the sooner it will stop!

If, however, you feel your child really has a problem, go and discuss it with your GP or Health Visitor. There may be a good reason why he is bed wetting. Don't forget that even if you don't know your Health Visitor very well, or at all, she will always come and discuss any particular problems you are having with your child.

Occasionally boys at puberty have what are called 'wet dreams'. These happen when he masturbates or ejaculates in his sleep. This is a normal part of growing up and should not be confused with wetting the bed. The child may feel embarrassed about it but just try not to notice! If you feel comfortable enough to do so, it is quite a good idea to warn your son that this might happen and that it is nothing to worry about – in the same way that you might talk to your daughter about starting her periods. (See Chapter 24 on Pregnancy in Adolescence.)

BITES

Dog bites

Every year 56,000 children are bitten badly enough by dogs for their parents to think they need hospital treatment. Out of those, 25,000 are bitten at home. These figures should be enough to make us all think more seriously about man's (and child's) best friend.

I am not knocking having a dog. We have a dog too, and she is very much a part of all of our lives, but perhaps we all need to be more aware of the down-side of having a pet – especially if you have very young children.

Children should never be left alone with a strange dog, or dogs. Dogs have a pack instinct, and if one of them attacks there is a possibility they all will. Always teach a child to be cautious with other people's dogs. They must NOT approach a strange dog.

Parents should be on their guard if a dog does not show any respect for a child or does not look him in the eye.

If a dog attacks your child it will almost certainly snap, bite and let go. According to the RSPCA it is rare for a dog to hang on – but don't depend on this as some breeds don't let go. The bite may be little more than a scratch or it may be very serious. Dogs, like humans, carry germs in their mouths. They have sharp, pointed teeth and when they bite these germs are driven deep into the child's flesh. The child may be bleeding and in severe cases his face, arms, hands or legs may be badly damaged.

WHAT TO DO

● The main thing to do is to get the dog away from the child as quickly as you can. The RSPCA suggests that you grab a broom handle or a dust-bin lid in order to shield yourself from the dog while you get the child to a safe place. If possible, lock up the dog in a room or shed and call the RSPCA. They recommend that any dog which has bitten once could bite again and should be put down, harsh though that sounds.

● ANY *dog bite needs urgent medical attention.* The child may be very shocked and this must be treated along with his injuries (see Chapter 27 on Shock).

> ## REMEMBER – SHOCK LOOKS LIKE THIS
>
> - His face may be very pale and grey-looking
> - His skin may feel cold and clammy
> - His pulse may feel fast and weak
> - He may be frightened and fidgety
> - He may be very thirsty
> - He may yawn and 'gasp' for air
> - He may say everything feels fuzzy
> - He may become unconscious

There are two sorts of bites: those which only scratch the surface of the skin and deep ones which cause serious injury.

For 'surface' bites

- Wash the area around the bite with warm, soapy water for about five minutes – this is to make quite sure that any germs the dog might have transferred onto the skin have been washed away.

- Dry the skin and cover the bite with a clean dressing.

- Take the child to a doctor – who will want to know if the child is up to date with his immunisations, which include tetanus. This is *the* important injection to protect a child who has been bitten or scratched by a dog (or cat). (Tetanus, or lock-jaw, is a disease of the nervous system which, among other things, causes the spine, the neck and the jaw to go into spasm, and the child may die. You rarely see it now because of immunisation, which is given to all babies who attend either the child health clinic or the baby clinic run by the GP or Health Visitor.) The doctor may also prescribe antibiotics.

For 'deep' bites

- The child will be terrified. Comfort and reassure him. Tell him the dog is now out of the way and *cannot* get out – as long as this is the case.

- Tell him what you are going to do before you do it.

- He will almost certainly be in shock. Lie him down and raise his legs – if they have not been injured (see Chapter 27 on Shock).

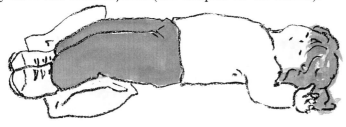

> ### REMEMBER – SHOCK LOOKS LIKE THIS
>
> - His face may be very pale and grey-looking
> - His skin may feel cold and clammy
> - His pulse may feel fast and weak
> - He may be frightened and fidgety
> - He may be very thirsty
> - He may yawn and 'gasp' for air
> - He may say everything feels fuzzy
> - He may become unconscious

- If he starts to be sick or to become unconscious, roll him quickly over into the Recovery Position.

- If he becomes unconscious, open his airway and check his breathing. If it stops, start your ABC Resuscitation Routine immediately.

> **A** for **AIRWAY** (is it clear?)
>
> **B** for **BREATHING** (is he breathing?)
>
> **C** for **CIRCULATION** (is his heart beating?)

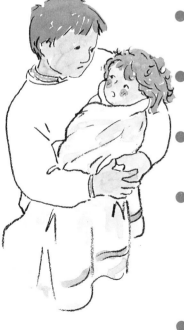

- If, however, he is breathing normally, put direct pressure onto the wounds. This will help to stop the bleeding (see Chapter 6 on Bleeding).

- Do not let the child rub or touch any face wounds, especially if his eye is injured. You may have to wrap his arms inside a blanket if he is too small to understand that he mustn't touch.

- In very bad cases the limb may even be torn. You must support this as best you can until the ambulance arrives; but the most important thing is to stop the bleeding.

- The dog may have actually bitten off the child's finger (or toe). This may sound unthinkable, but if it does happen you must be prepared to pick it up – if it is still around – and put it in a plastic bag (preferably with some ice), then label it with the child's *name, age and the time and date of the accident.* You must make sure it gets to the hospital *at the same time as the child* – there is then a good chance that it may be sewn back in place.

- Put clean, dry dressings on the wounds and bandage them firmly in place.

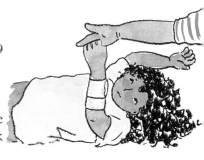

- Lift up the hand or leg that has been bitten.

- Call for an ambulance, if you haven't already done so, by dialling 999 and tell them what has happened.

Human bites

All bites are serious because the germs that are naturally kept in the mouths of all animals (including humans) are 'injected' as the teeth sink into the flesh and the muscles and structures beneath it.

When a human bites a human, it tends to be rather worse than an animal bite because the teeth crush the tissues rather than piercing them.

Human bites, like other animal bites (and scratches), need to be taken seriously as far as the risk of tetanus is concerned. If your child has had the tetanus vaccine, which is normally included in his immunisation programme – given at his local clinic or doctor's surgery – then he will be protected and you don't have to worry.

It is worth double-checking that this has been done. (Sometimes, for instance, if a child is newly arrived in this country, he may well *not* be covered by the tetanus vaccine, in which case this will be part of his medical treatment, once he registers with a doctor.)

If you see unexplained bites either on your child or a child you are looking after, you should tell someone about them.

If you are the parent, talk to your child about how he thinks he got the 'marks' on his body. Don't say immediately that you recognise them as bites – they may not be anyway. He may be pleased to talk about them and there may be some simple explanation, or he may find it difficult to tell you, in which case try not to push him. He may not be ready to talk to you but make sure he realises that you are ready to listen to him whenever he wants.

You might want to go and talk to the teacher in case the child is being bullied, or you might find it easier to go and talk to your Health Visitor or doctor.

If you are a teacher or carer you might start by telling the parents about the marks and that you are concerned. However, if you continue to see them and if you feel for some reason the parent is not taking the situation seriously enough, then call your local doctor or have a chat with the Health Visitor.

There may be some simple explanation or it may be that the child is being bullied. There is also the possibility that the child is being abused by someone looking after him.

If you are a parent and you are worried that *you may be harming your child in this, or any other way*, and you feel you would like to talk to other parents who have had similar difficulties, you might like to talk to Parentline.

Parentline is run by parents for parents. It is a twenty-four-hour service (after 5 p.m. there is an answerphone which will tell you the telephone number of a volunteer you can speak to). There are twenty-five branches throughout the country. If there isn't one in your town, you can ring this central number for your nearest branch. The telephone number is:

Parentline 0268 757077

If you feel that a troubled child you know might like to talk to someone *in total confidence* on the telephone, he should ring Childline. This is a free twenty-four-hour service. The switchboard operator will transfer him to a trained counsellor. It is sometimes difficult to get through to Childline because so many children phone in, but he *will* get through eventually. The Freefone telephone number is:

Childline 0800 1111

OR the child might like to write in confidence to:

Childline
Freepost 1111, London N1 0BR (no stamp needed).

If for any reason you are worried about a child you know who you think might be being ill-treated by being bitten, or in any other way, or perhaps *you* were treated in this way as a child and would like to talk about it, you might like to contact a new organisation set up by the NSPCC, called the NSPCC Child Protection Helpline. It is a twenty-four hour *confidential* counselling service run by qualified social workers for anyone who may want to get help or ask advice about any sort of child abuse. The Freefone telephone number is:

NSPCC Child Protection Helpline 0800 800 500

The NSPCC also has a helpful leaflet for parents and carers called *Protect Your Child*. You can send for it to this address:

NSPCC
67 Saffron Hill, London EC1N 8RS.

You can also go to your local Social Services Department (address in telephone directory). Don't hesitate to ask them if you can have a confidential chat with a social worker – they are trained to deal with these sorts of problems. Social workers are bound *by law* to help in any way they can with a child who may be being badly treated.

Snake bites

Snake bites are rarely fatal in Great Britain where the only poisonous snakes are adders. However, those people who keep snakes as pets occasionally lose them – they just decide to go walkabout or should I say 'slitherabout'! Occasionally pet snakes attack their owners.

Snake bites are most unpleasant, because it is difficult to know how poisonous the venom is – this is liquid they squirt into you when they bite you. Your reaction to the bite could quite often make the child feel very frightened and may even cause severe shock.

When you are travelling abroad it is important for you to know that some countries have many sorts of poisonous and dangerous snakes. These may be difficult to recognise, particularly if you are visitors to the country. However, it is very important to be able to recognise the snake that bit your child so that the right anti-venom (anti-poison) serum can be given.

Be aware of how important this is and try to make a note, at least mentally, of what the snake looked like – its colour and markings are the best things to remember, as well as where it bit your child. If, of course, you have been brave (or stupid) enough to have captured or killed it, keep it so that the experts can tell exactly which kind of snake it was. *Don't forget to take it with you when you take your child to hospital.*

WHAT TO LOOK FOR

If your child has been bitten by a snake:

- He may feel a bit woozy and he may not be able to 'see straight'.

- He may feel sick or actually *be* sick.

- You may be able to see one or two puncture wounds – like needle pricks. These may be very painful and the area around them will be red and swollen.

- He may want to spit a lot and will seem to have a lot of saliva in and around his mouth – this may be because he is feeling sick or, more seriously, it may be a later stage of 'venom reaction' which shows that the poison from the snake bite has got into his blood stream and his body is reacting to that. If this is happening he will almost certainly be sweating a lot.

- He will almost certainly be shocked (see Chapter 27 on Shock).

REMEMBER – SHOCK LOOKS LIKE THIS

- His face may be very pale and grey-looking
- His skin may feel cold and clammy
- His pulse may feel fast and weak
- He may be frightened and fidgety
- He may be very thirsty
- He may yawn and 'gasp' for air
- He may say everything feels fuzzy
- He may become unconscious

199

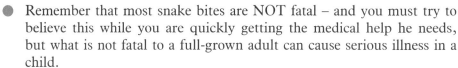

WHAT TO DO

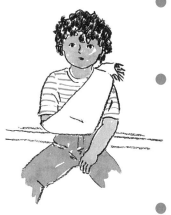

● This child will be terrified and probably so will you. Try not to show him how you feel, but deal with it as calmly as you can. Reassure him as much as possible.

● Remember that most snake bites are NOT fatal – and you must try to believe this while you are quickly getting the medical help he needs, but what is not fatal to a full-grown adult can cause serious illness in a child.

● Try to keep him as still as you can. If the snake has bitten him on his arm, for instance, you need to keep the arm as still as possible. It will help to bandage the arm to his chest, keeping it below the level of his heart, to try to stop the poison being pumped by the heart around his body.

   If he has been bitten on his leg, bandage it to the other leg to stop him from moving it.

● You will need medical help urgently. If the accident has happened in the UK, call for an ambulance by dialling 999 and tell them exactly what has happened. If you saw the snake, try to describe it as accurately as you can.

   (If you are in a foreign country you will want to get the child to hospital quickly – a taxi is probably the quickest route, if you don't know how to call for an ambulance. It is always useful, if you go away with children, to learn a few vital words of the language of the country you are visiting, even if you don't speak it well. You might want to know how to say, 'I have a sick child', 'Take me to the doctor/hospital', 'This is an emergency' and so on.)

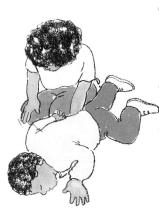

● If you have time, wash the area around the bite carefully with plenty of warm, soapy water, if that is possible, but if it means moving him a lot, don't do it. Just leave him, reassure him and tell him that help is on the way.

● If you feel he is going to be sick, put him in the Recovery Position, but watch him carefully.

● If, however, his breathing becomes difficult, check his airway and be prepared to start your ABC Resuscitation Routine immediately (see Chapter 3 on ABC Resuscitation Routine).

A for **AIRWAY**   (is it clear?)

B for **BREATHING**   (is he breathing?)

C for **CIRCULATION**   (is his heart beating?)

BOILS AND ABSCESSES

These are large infected spots, often starting from a very minor injury to the skin which has got dirty and has then been neglected. They can be very nasty and if they are not seen to can cause the infection to spread into the blood. If this happens the child could die.

So, abscesses and boils must be taken seriously.

WHAT TO LOOK FOR

- The area around the boil (abscess) will be red, and swollen.

- It will be very painful to the touch.

- Sometimes there are small red lines leading from the area out onto the surrounding skin. This is a serious sign and means that the infection is beginning to spread.

WHAT TO DO

- The child needs to see a doctor as soon as possible. If the boil or abscess is just red and painful he will advise you to do one of two things that will quickly bring the boil or abscess to a head – the quicker you do this, the faster you can help the pain. The doctor will tell you either to 'hot-spoon' bathe it, or to put some special paste onto it. Both of these do the same sort of job.

- Once the infection has reached a head, the doctor will probably lance it. This means nicking it with a small scalpel blade. As he does so, the pus will ooze out and the pain will ease.

- The doctor will prescribe antibiotics to make sure that the infection is cleared completely from the child's body. (He must take ALL of the medicine, so that he doesn't build up an immunity against it – this is important and is the only way to make sure that the antibiotics work every time he needs to take them.)

BREATH HOLDING

This is an alarming situation for parents of young children to deal with. It usually happens during a temper tantrum or if a child has had an accident and is in a lot of pain.

Just be aware that a child will be as frightened and shocked as you are by the strength of his anger. This needs super-human qualities from you not to get too involved with what is happening and you must stay

201

as calm as you can – even though this will seem to be almost impossible to do sometimes.

Temper tantrums

These usually happen when *you* want to do one thing and the child doesn't – rushing, for example, so try to allow a little more time for any shenanigans.

If you and your child clash about putting on a coat or getting in the buggy, for instance, try to head it off by taking those things with you, rather than insisting at the time that he puts it on or gets into it.

It is important that whatever the argument between you is about – even if it does end up with him holding his breath – you don't give in at the end of it. He must learn, however hard it is for him – and you – that although you realise he is angry, he cannot and must not behave in this way. The message is this is NOT the way to get what he wants in future.

If you don't make this clear after the first episode, it will get worse and he may do it every time things are not going his way.

There is no use trying to reason with a child who is having a temper tantrum and is at breath-holding stage. He cannot see or hear you clearly enough to be able to communicate with you – or you with him.

Once a child starts to hold his breath his face will go red with anger to blue or 'blotchy' grey. There is a possibility he could fit, although this is rare, or, more likely, he might faint.

As soon as he 'lets go', by losing consciousness, his normal breathing will return. On its own, therefore, breath holding is not dangerous. The danger is that he may injure himself before that stage. Make sure he is safe by seeing that there is nothing around on which he can hurt himself and nothing that he can knock his head on if it looks as though he is going to keel over.

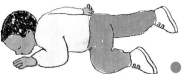

WHAT TO DO

● If he does lose consciousness put him in the Recovery Position.

● Once he comes around, which will be almost immediately, cuddle and reassure him. He will probably be exhausted so it is a good idea to tuck him up and let him have a sleep – if you are not in the supermarket at the time, in which case just pack him into the car and go. (You will probably be glad to get out of there anyway.) Other than that try not to make too much of it. He must *not* be aware that you have been at all put out by this episode. And if you have been – you just have to ACT.

● *If he has a fit, go with his movements* – don't try to stop him. Once the fit has started it will take on a 'life' of its own. It will probably be very short and as soon as he starts breathing normally again, roll him into the Recovery Position (see Chapter 17 on Fits). This, however, will be very upsetting for you – particularly if you have had an argument with him – but try not to show him how upset you are. He may wet or soil himself during a fit, so be aware that this might happen and don't make too much of it.

● *If your child holds his breath after being hurt in an accident* and if he loses consciousness, roll him over into the Recovery Position.

Once he is breathing normally you can deal with his injuries. Stop any bleeding by direct pressure to the cuts. Cover them as soon as you can with a clean, dry dressing (see Chapter 6 on Bleeding).

● If he has burnt himself, cool the burn with cold water as quickly as you can (see Chapter 7 on Burns and Scalds).

For other injuries, see the chapter under the heading of the injury.

● If you feel the child has injured himself badly phone your doctor, or in an emergency call for an ambulance by dialling 999.

● If your child holds his breath a lot, it might be helpful to talk it through with your Health Visitor or your doctor.

COUGHS AND COLDS

Coughs and colds are not by themselves at all dangerous. But parents should be aware that small babies with infections of their upper breathing passages should be watched very carefully. (Doctors call these infections URTI, which stands for Upper Respiratory Tract Infections.)

The breathing and hearing system is made up of a complex series of passages leading from the ears and nose down to the voice box. The swallowing and breathing passages, leading to the stomach and lungs, complete the system (see Chapter 2 on How the Body Works).

Any of these passages can become inflamed and swollen with an infection which may start as an ordinary cold or cough. It is often difficult to tell with a baby or young child exactly what is the matter. Sometimes a child will pull on one or both ears and scream with pain – this *may* be earache. Alternatively, the child could be teething. Try to treat coughs and colds by what you think you see.

If a baby or a very young child has a temperature over 39°C (102°F), always take him to see the doctor. You can never be sure what is brewing.

A blocked-up nose can be unpleasant, in a baby especially, or if the child is a thumb-sucker. There are several ways you might be able to help to make him feel better.

WHAT TO DO

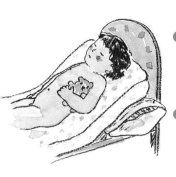

● Tilt the head-end of the baby's mattress by putting a pillow or two *underneath* it. This allows the trapped mucus in the nose to drain downwards and to clear. NEVER put a pillow directly under a young child's head – he could suffocate, particularly if he is snuffly.

● Humidify the atmosphere by putting moisture into the air artificially – any heating dries out the air. You may want to buy a steam vaporiser if you have a child who is often snuffly, especially if any of your children get croup (see below and Chapter 10 on Croup).

● Give the child a 'decongestant' to breathe. My favourites are the ones which you sprinkle on the sheet or on his pyjamas (mind his eyes), or the good old menthol rub which you rub on the chest before the child goes to sleep. Any of these will help the child to feel less bunged up. However, DO NOT USE THESE FOR SMALL BABIES – the vapour could make the child unconscious.

● Use nose-drops to loosen the mucus. Ask your pharmacist to make you up some Normal Saline (salt and water) nose-drops. If the cold is very bad – perhaps it is stopping the baby from feeding or sleeping – ask your doctor for some decongestant nose-drops to thin down the sticky mucus in the nose and make it easier for the child to breathe.

● Sometimes a very snuffly child needs a sedative to help him sleep through the night. If he *hasn't* got a temperature, try homoeopathic camomile drops. They are calming and soothing and extremely effective, particularly if the child is teething. Snuffly noses often go with teething, for no obvious reason.

● There are other very good homoeopathic remedies which you can buy for coughs and colds. These are explained in a leaflet you can get at your chemist (if he sells homoeopathic remedies) or see a homoeopath.

● If the child is obviously poorly and has a temperature he may need a drug to bring his temperature down. The best sort is a paracetamol-syrup (some are sugar, colour *and glycerine*★ free). Remember not to use aspirin-based products for children under twelve.

● Try to keep a child with a cold in bed, or at least off school or kindergarten – there is no place like home for a sickly child. This will be difficult if you are working, but worth bearing in mind. Children get better much more quickly if they have one or two days indoors.

Vaporisers, either manual or electric, can be purchased from most big chemists. The prices range (at the time of writing) from about £10 for the candle-lit one (manual but fiddly) to between £20 and £95 for an

★no animal products.

204

electric one. They are all tested for safety. The £95 one gives you steam control – you can have as much or as little as you need. All the electric ones have the choice of hot or cold steam.

If you are unable to find a vapouriser in chemists near you, you can buy them from:

John Bell and Croyden
50 Wigmore Street, London W1.
Tel. 071 935 5555
If you cannot call at the shop they will send it to you by mail order.

CUTS AND BRUISES

Children fall over a lot – it is part of growing up and learning what they can and cannot do. Most children will have bruises at some point in their lives, usually on their shins or knees, and many will have cuts or grazes from time to time (see Chapter 6 on Bleeding). They don't, however, normally fall on their faces or on their trunks (the upper part of the body). If you see a child who has these types of bruises or cuts, he may be being bullied or being hit by an adult.

It is important not to ignore a child with these sort of injuries, especially if you notice them on more than one occasion. You must try and protect this child and find out what has been happening. If he is not your child you may want to tell the school or the Health Visitor. Whatever you do or whoever you tell, DON'T pretend that you haven't seen it.

WHAT TO DO

- If the child just grazes himself, the tiny amount of blood around the wound clots. It is a good idea to wash it gently with cool water, particularly if the graze is very dirty. A graze will usually heal by itself, but if it carries on bleeding, a sticky plaster will help protect it. Try to use one which isn't waterproof. These tend to make the skin underneath the plaster sweat and stop the wound from healing as well as it could.

- Leave the plaster on for a day or two – and no more – then gently but firmly peel it off (the bath is the best place to do this). If the child is left with a black mark where the plaster was, it should easily wear off. If it is really unsightly, you may want to remove it with plaster remover from the chemist's, but be careful – if this gets into the wound, even though it is semi-healed it will sting.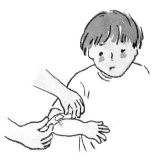

  (If your child's skin starts to redden or swell up around the plaster it probably means that he is allergic to the sticky part of the sticking plaster. Try to use a low-allergy or 'micropore' sort instead.)

● Some children get very upset when they do anything to their bodies, even though we know 'it's only a graze'. Generally speaking a cuddle will put it right and I must admit that this is one of the times I use sweets to distract attention. It usually works!

Bruising is bleeding into the tissues underneath the skin. If the child has an accident, say he falls off his bicycle, he may have lots of bruises and may be extremely shocked. Always be aware of the possibility of shock, even if the child hasn't broken anything or there isn't any blood to see (see Chapter 27 on Shock).

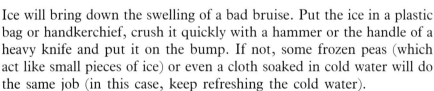

REMEMBER – SHOCK LOOKS LIKE THIS

- ● His face may be very pale and grey-looking
- ● His skin may feel cold and clammy
- ● His pulse may feel fast and weak
- ● He may be frightened and fidgety
- ● He may be very thirsty
- ● He may yawn and 'gasp' for air
- ● He may say everything feels fuzzy
- ● He may become unconscious

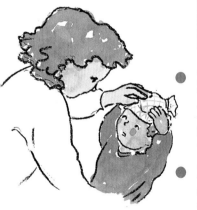

● Ice will bring down the swelling of a bad bruise. Put the ice in a plastic bag or handkerchief, crush it quickly with a hammer or the handle of a heavy knife and put it on the bump. If not, some frozen peas (which act like small pieces of ice) or even a cloth soaked in cold water will do the same job (in this case, keep refreshing the cold water).

● Homoeopathic arnica cream, rubbed gently into a bruised area, helps to stop the bruising and soothes the pain. If it is a bad bump arnica pills melted on the tongue will help as well – remember, all homoeopathic remedies are safe for children but if in doubt, consult a homoeopath.

EAR ACHE

Ear ache in children is very common. It is caused by an infection of the middle ear and if you ignore it or don't recognise what is happening, the infection can spread inwards to the brain. It is important to get any child with an ear ache to the doctor, or the doctor to the child, quickly.

Middle ear infection often follows a cold, sore throat or any infection of the breathing or swallowing passages. The child wakes up (it often happens at night) screaming and usually with a high temperature. He may or may not be pulling at his ears. He will be in a lot of pain. An older child will be able to tell you what is the matter; a younger one, or a baby, won't.

WHAT TO DO

- *Don't put anything into a child's ear*, oil or drops, for instance, without having talked to your doctor first. It may just hide the symptoms and in some cases may be dangerous.

- Call the doctor, no matter what time of the night it is, if you think the child has an ear infection. If you are wrong he, or she, will understand.

- The best treatment for ear infection is usually antibiotics. Occasionally, when the doctor looks in the ear through his 'auroscope' he may see that the ear-drum is *not* inflamed – in other words there is no infection – and yet the child may still be complaining of ear ache. If the nose is blocked, he may give you some nose-drops to thin down the mucus in the nose. Mucus may be pressing on the tube leading from the nose to the ear and causing the pain (see Chapter 2 on How the Body Works).

Objects pushed into the ear

Children like to play with their ears – they feel nice, and when they poke things into them they tickle; they may even make a nice noise when an object goes in and out. Unfortunately one of two things may happen. Either on one of the journeys into the ear the thing that is being pushed or pulled – commonly a cotton bud, hair-grip or slide – punctures the drum, or – if it is a small enough object such as a bead, Lego brick or button – it may just get stuck. You may not know for some time afterwards that the child has done either of these things, particularly with a little child.

The first clue you may get is that you may see a sticky discharge coming from the child's ear or on his pillow, or you may find him pulling at his ear because he has a 'blocked feeling' in it. He may, of course, just be in a lot of pain.

- If you feel that your child may have pushed an object into his ear, or you feel that he has something wrong with his ear (perhaps he keeps fiddling with it – or he may not have been himself for a while), *take him to the doctor.*

- When the doctor looks in the child's ear with an auroscope he will check for injury to the ear-drum and will probably see the object. The child will almost certainly need antibiotics in case he gets an infection.

- DO NOT in any circumstances probe into the ear or try to remove the object yourself – even if you can see it when you have a look. All you will do is to push it further in. It will then be much more difficult to get it out.

207

- Don't delay in getting medical help. If there is something stuck in his ear and it is left for too long, he could end up being deaf in that ear.

If an insect flies inside the ear

This is an extremely unpleasant experience for the child – some children become totally hysterical. Remember, the buzzing noise is magnified many times inside the ear.

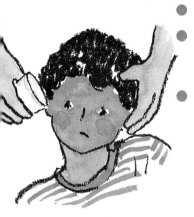

- You must comfort and reassure the child.

- If he is sensible and old enough, you may be able to trickle water into the ear to wash the insect out – a jug or a lipped cup, with luke-warm water (not warm, not cold) will probably do the trick.

- If the child is hysterical, especially a younger child, a drop of eau-de-cologne, lavender water or after-shave dropped into the ear will kill the insect instantly. To do this, the child has to be held very still so that the liquid doesn't splash into the eyes. Wrapping the child up inside a blanket or towel will keep his arms out of the way and help you reach the ear easily. The child will need a lot of comforting.

   You need to get him to hospital as soon as you can.

Other things to be aware of

- *If the child has had a 'grommets' operation* DO NOT put anything IN THE EAR, not even water. This is an operation given to young children who have 'glue ear'. The 'glue' is a build-up of sticky fluid behind the ear-drum; often the only clue parents get that this is happening is if the child cannot hear or speak properly (because he isn't *hearing* any speech).

   Grommets are small, plastic tubes which are placed through a small slit made in the child's ear-drum, under a general anaesthetic. These will help this 'glue' drain out. The grommets, having done their job, usually fall out by themselves over the next year to eighteen months.

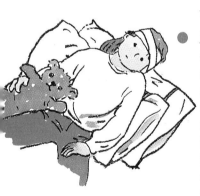

- *If your child has any discharge* coming from his ear – including blood, clear fluid or pus – he must see a doctor immediately. The blood or clear fluid could mean an injury to the skull or brain and the pus could mean an ear infection. They are all serious in their own way and must not be ignored. If you think your child may have an injury like this you may not want to move him. He will probably be frightened and in pain. Reassure and comfort him, then cover the bad ear gently with a sterile (or very clean) pad and bandage loosely around his head. Lie the child on the floor or bed, with the bad ear facing downwards. Call for an ambulance by dialling 999. Tell them what you think has happened. (See Chapter 19 on Head Injuries.)

- *When you are cleaning a child's ears* never poke anything down them, such as a cotton bud, to clean inside. Washing the whole ear area with a face cloth and plenty of soapy water is generally enough. If you see some brown, waxy stuff in the little hole, just wipe it gently away with the tip of your finger under the face cloth on the outside only. Do not poke – you can really damage the ear this way.

- *If your child suffers from 'blocked ears' on an aeroplane or at high altitude, the best way to clear the blockage is by yawning.* Swallowing also helps. Try whatever works for your child. Once the plane has reached a certain height the pain stops, so the important thing is to try to take his mind off it until then.

FAINTING

Children faint for all sorts of reasons, often to do with heat – either from the atmosphere when the weather or a room is too hot, or from inside their bodies when they develop a high temperature.

If a child faints he becomes unconscious for that brief moment, even though the moment he 'lies down' or falls to the floor he will usually recover. This is because as he hits the floor, the blood – which has for a second or two drained away from his brain – begins to flow back and he becomes conscious again. That is why you must always lie a child down who feels faint. NEVER try sitting a fainting child up in a chair even with his head down. HIS BODY NEEDS TO LIE DOWN – let it.

WHAT TO DO

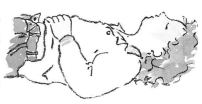

- Once he is on the floor, make sure his airway is open and that there is no tight clothing, either at his neck or waist, that will make it difficult for him to breathe.

- If he starts to make choking sounds as if he is going to be sick roll him quickly over into the Recovery Position.

- When he starts to come round, comfort and reassure him. Even if he is still feeling decidedly off-colour he will be comforted by knowing you are there.

- If the child does not come round quickly, check his airway and breathing. If you feel he may be unconscious or if he does not come round easily, then open his airway and be prepared to start your ABC Resuscitation Routine.

> **A** for **AIRWAY** (is it clear?)
>
> **B** for **BREATHING** (is he breathing?)
>
> **C** for **CIRCULATION** (is his heart beating?)

- Check the child for any injury.

- If the child is unconscious rather than having fainted, he needs to be seen urgently in hospital. Call for an ambulance by dialling 999 and tell them what has happened.

If a child faints on more than one occasion he should be seen by a doctor to check if there is any serious medical reason why this is happening. He may faint if he doesn't eat regularly or when he has to do something which he finds stressful, or he may have a minor form of epilepsy (see Chapter 17 on Fits). Any of these situations need to be investigated.

FEVER

There is only one way you can tell if a child has a high fever and that is to take his temperature with a thermometer. There are various sorts you can buy – the most useful is a plastic strip that you put on the child's forehead. Even though this is not the most accurate thermometer, you can get a good idea if the child has a high temperature by how quickly it moves up the scale. I find that thermometers you put under a child's arm are less useful – the child usually wriggles so much that although it should be more accurate, it rarely is (and there is a danger that it might break). A digital thermometer is one you put in the child's mouth and it beeps at a certain temperature – the only disadvantage is that it is twice the price of either of the others.

WHAT TO LOOK FOR

- Usually a child with a temperature will go off his food.

- Children particularly look 'feverish'. They usually have red, hot cheeks and bright, almost staring eyes.

- He will be restless and unhappy, or he may just be miserable and sleep a lot.

You cannot ignore a child with a temperature, especially a high one. You have to bring it down somehow, quickly and calmly.

Sometimes a child's temperature will start at say 38°C (100°F) and will slowly creep up the thermometer. In a minor illness, such as a cold, it may even stay where it is.

WHAT TO DO

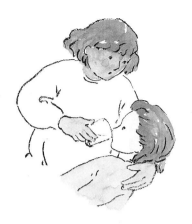

If your child has a slight temperature

- Try to encourage him to drink, the more he drinks the quicker his temperature will come down. Water is best – try to keep off fizzy or sweet drinks as they might make him sick.

- If he is hot and sticky, encourage him to have a bath or sponge his body down with tepid (not warm, not cold) water.

- Take his night-clothes off and cover him with a light sheet.

Some babies and young children, however, have extremely unstable temperatures. One minute they are at 38°C (100°F) and the next at 41°C (106°F) – especially if the child is crying. Crying tends to push the temperature up in an already feverish child. These are the children you have to watch as they can have a fit (see Chapter 17 on Fits). The awful thing is that you never know which of your children is going to fit – unless they have done so before and you know what to expect.

If your child has a high temperature

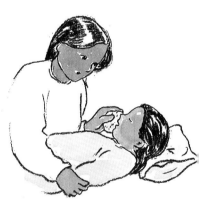

- Give the child some paracetamol-syrup. The dose needed will be written clearly on the bottle. (You can get ones that are low/no sugar with no colour agents.) This will immediately start to tackle the temperature. Never give more than the dose or more frequently than recommended on the bottle.

- Wash the child with tepid (not warm, not cold) water or give him a bath. Leave his skin slightly damp after drying.

- Take his temperature again. If it shows no sign of coming down, put on an electric fan (or a fan heater on cold), and place it near to the child's body. (Make sure it is not near enough for the child to touch.) Or open a window in the child's room, but not one directly over him. This may seem drastic but it is an effective way of bringing a high temperature down.

- Children with high temperatures get frightened and may have nightmares. It is important to reassure him and comfort him but not necessarily to *cuddle* him. Tell him, if he is old enough to understand, that when his temperature is very high it would make him hotter to have a cuddle. See if he will settle for a story or game instead.

- If you are worried CALL THE DOCTOR, especially for a baby or very young child.

211

FISH HOOKS

Doctors are reporting seeing more and more children with fish hooks well and truly stuck into various bits of them. If you can get to a doctor quickly do so, rather than trying to get the fish hook out yourself. If not, the following technique, picked up from South Australian fishermen, will show you how to get the hook out:

WHAT TO DO

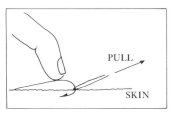

- Reassure the child. He will be frightened and unsure what you are going to try and do.

- Lie him down before you begin, in case he feels faint.

- Loop a piece of string around the hook and wrap the free ends around your index finger.

- Hold the hook between the thumb and index finger of the other hand and press down slightly to allow the hook to slide out from under the skin.

- Slowly pull the string tight in line with the shaft of the hook and give the string a sharp sudden pull.

OR you can use the following technique preferred by English fly-fishermen. This involves parents who fish with their children (and by themselves) carrying a small pair of wire cutters or pliers with them in their tackle box.

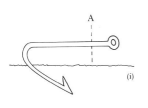

- Cut the hook at 'A' using wire-cutters or pliers.

- Feed the hook back out through the skin as shown.

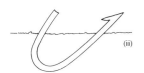

If you can't get the fish hook out, or you don't feel like doing this yourself, take the child to a doctor as soon as you can.

After using either of these methods you must wash the child's skin with soap and water or use one of the handy sachets in your first aid kit. (See pages 281-283 on 'First Aid Kit'.) Then cover with a sticky plaster. Always make sure that your child is up-to-date with his tetanus injections.

LICE AND NITS

It is most parents' dread to find lice or nits (the eggs the louse lays) in their child's hair or, worse, to get a letter from school saying the child has lice or nits! It's as if somewhere along the line we have failed (again) as parents. In fact most children today, whichever school or kindergarten they go to, will be in contact with a child with nits – but with luck and a few precautions they may avoid catching them. The louse prefers clean heads, especially girls with short dark hair (boys rarely get lice and nits).

Little children are more likely to get them because they put their heads together more. The louse moves from one head onto another by swinging along the hair. The only way lice can get from one head to the next is if two children are so close to each other that their hair is actually touching – not an unusual situation in young children. And you can't stop children from cuddling or being close to each other!

The louse looks like a little money spider – no bigger than a matchhead and much smaller if it is a baby louse. *It can only live in the hair.* Once it leaves the head, it dies. Lice feed by making pin pricks in the scalp and sucking up the blood. It is this action that causes the itching, not the insects crawling about the hair, and that might be the first sign that your child has lice. Unfortunately they may have been there for quite some time before the itching starts and may have laid many eggs (nits) on the hair before the infestation is discovered.

The eggs the louse lays on the hair are flesh-coloured (the white ones are the egg shells). Each egg is oval-shaped and is about the size of a pin head. They stick onto the hair with a special kind of cement and are impossible to remove – this was how superglue was invented! The only way to get them out is by using a special lotion (*not* the shampoo) which kills the lice and penetrates the eggs. However, if it is not used properly, or there is a second infestation within a fairly short period, it may not work as well the next time. In other words the child becomes 'immune' to the lotion (in exactly the same way as if antibiotics are not used properly; the antibiotic that worked well before may not work on the new infection and the doctor may have to prescribe a different, possibly stronger drug).

Every few months the head lotion is changed and you will have to ask your pharmacist which is the one that is currently being used. The ones presently in use contain malathion, carbaryl, phenothrin or permethrin.

Children don't really enjoy having this lotion put on because it is unpleasant. It feels cold – that's because it has an alcohol base – it stinks and they have to let it dry naturally and then leave it on their hair overnight. The most important thing is not to splash it into the child's eyes accidentally – ask her to hold a cloth over her face while it is being put on the hair. Once the lotion hits the hair the lice just fall out, so it's

213

best to sit with a towel around her shoulders.

Once she has got the lotion on the hair she mustn't wash her hair for twelve hours or swim for two weeks – the chlorine in the pool lessens the effect. If the head feels a little itchy afterwards it is probably because the alcohol in the lotion has dried out the scalp. A little oil or conditioner on her scalp will help.

Don't bother to remove the dead eggs. Nit combing with one of those special combs is both painful and unnecessary and it may put children off from telling you that they have an itchy head in the future. If they look a bit unsightly, a drop of vinegar in the rinsing water will loosen them sufficiently for them to be combed (with an ordinary comb) or washed out.

If you have a child who often gets lice and nits, you may be interested in a new product just on the market. This will, according to the manufacturers, stop the child getting lice if it is sprayed on the hair three times a week before school. They describe it as 'the first and only user-friendly, pump-action, louse repellent spray'!

There are other ways that you can prevent your child from getting lice, although these may not always be fool-proof.

- If your child has long hair it is easier for a louse to swing onto the loose hair that may be falling over her shoulders – try to persuade your child to tie it back.

- Comb your child's hair through every night – or as often as possible – with as fine a comb as you can. The louse may not lay its eggs right away and if you can comb it out quickly, it may not have a chance to do so.

- Check the child's hair regularly. The louse has favourite places – usually the warmest – to start its family and these should be checked first. They are: behind the ears, under the hair at the nape of the neck and on the crown of the head.

But remember, if you child does get lice and nits, it's not the end of the world. If you over-react it can make her feel very guilty and, after all, it's not her fault!

NOSE-BLEEDS

Nose-bleeds are very common in children, particularly in hot weather. Although they are bloody and messy, they are rarely serious and it is not usually necessary for the child to see a doctor unless the nose-bleed continues for over half an hour or *the child has just had a bad fall* or crack on the head. A bleeding nose, particularly if the blood is mixed with clear fluid, might suggest that the child's skull is fractured. This needs urgent medical attention (see Chapter 19 on Head Injuries).

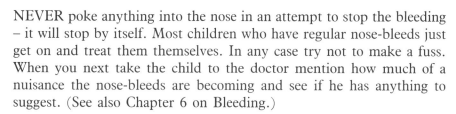

WHAT TO DO

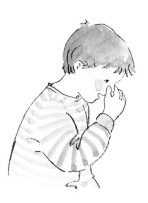

For a simple nose-bleed

- Sit the child forward and let the blood drip away. Pinch the soft part of the nose above the nostrils – an older child can do this himself.

- Tell him not to talk (impossible for some kids) and to try not to swallow, cough or sniff, or blow his nose.

- If it is a bad nose-bleed hold one or two cracked ice cubes in a plastic bag over the bridge of the nose. Ice helps the blood to clot quickly. If you have no ice a few frozen peas in a plastic bag will do the same job.

- In a bad nose-bleed keep up the pressure for ten minutes then check to see if it has stopped. If the bleeding has not stopped get medical help.

NEVER poke anything into the nose in an attempt to stop the bleeding – it will stop by itself. Most children who have regular nose-bleeds just get on and treat them themselves. In any case try not to make a fuss. When you next take the child to the doctor mention how much of a nuisance the nose-bleeds are becoming and see if he has anything to suggest. (See also Chapter 6 on Bleeding.)

Broken nose

If your child is playing a ball game and the ball is kicked or thrown straight into his face, and there is blood everywhere and his nose looks a funny shape, there is a good chance he has broken it.

If he has had any bump on the nose the thing to do is to reduce the swelling as quickly as possible with an ice-pack. Then if you think he may have broken the nose take him to hospital and they will X-ray it – this is the only way to find out. If you think the child has broken his nose, don't give him anything to eat or drink in case he needs an anaesthetic when he gets to hospital. More often than not, especially if the break is not causing breathing problems, you will be asked to bring him back to an ENT (Ear, Nose and Throat) clinic when the swelling has gone down.

Object stuck in the nose

Some children like to put things in any opening in their body, and noses are no exception. So any spare Lego bricks, small beads, coins, even upholstery foam may be stuck in a child's nostrils.

The danger is when you haven't noticed and he hasn't told you (toddlers rarely do) that something is there that shouldn't be. It may stay in the nose unnoticed for weeks.

The first clue you may get is a greenish, smelly discharge from one of his nostrils, or you may see that he is constantly rubbing or fiddling with his nose.

215

Even if you saw the child put something into his nose, *don't try and poke it to get it out*. You might push it further up. The child needs to go to hospital where they have special instruments to take these objects out of the nose. He may need to have an anaesthetic, so don't give him anything to eat or drink.

SORE THROATS

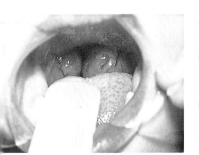

Tonsilitis. That is what a 'very sore throat' looks like. Sore! Sometimes you can see white patches on the tonsils or around the throat. This may mean that the infection is caused by streptococcus.

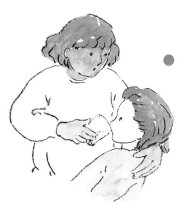

Most children have lots of sore throats, especially the kind where the tonsils are big, red and juicy. But in spite of what our mothers and grandmothers thought, tonsils are no longer automatically removed – no matter how large they are – because doctors now recognise they fight infection and help to protect a child from serious illness (see Chapter 2 on How the Body Works). In other words, tonsils fight any infection in the throat and try to stop it from reaching other parts of the breathing system. That is why it hurts so much when the child tries to swallow. The child might have a temperature if he has a sore throat.

WHAT TO DO

● The only help you can give to a baby or a very young child with a sore throat – they can't gargle – is paracetamol-syrup (try to use one that is colour- and sugar-free). This will bring any temperature down and take some of the pain away (see pages 210-211 on Fever).

● Give the child plenty of cold drinks – they will soothe his throat. If he is 'snuffly', help him to breathe more easily by humidifying the air (putting moisture back into it) or using a decongestant to thin down the sticky mucus in his nose (see pages 203-204 on Coughs and Colds).

There is one condition, however, that is more than a sore throat – it is an abscess of the tonsil, called quinsy.

You may think your child has this if he has a high temperature and won't or can't swallow because his throat hurts too much. He will be dribbling a lot and obviously in a lot of pain. He may not even want to open his mouth.

If you think that your child might have quinsy DO NOT give him anything to eat or drink. Take him immediately to the doctor or the hospital Accident and Emergency department. He will be given antibiotics and may have to have a small operation.

SPLINTERS AND PINS

These make prick marks in the skin and if you are not careful they can easily become infected.

WHAT TO DO

- If the child has got a splinter in his hand or foot (these are the most likely places) and you can see it, lift it out with tweezers, clean nails or fingertips. Grasp the splinter and pull it out in the opposite direction to the way it is lodged in the skin. Once the splinter is out, wash the area with soap and water. Dab a little disinfectant on it and cover with a plaster. Watch that the prick mark doesn't become infected. You can tell this if it becomes red, painful and sore, or if it develops a yellow pus-sy head.

- If you can't see a splinter because it is very small, clean the area with antiseptic, cover it and leave it. The splinter will drop out in its own time. Some doctors think that splinters are best left anyway.

- If the child has trodden on a pin and you can't get it out with a swift pull – leave it, pad around it with clean cotton wool and bandage over the padding so that it doesn't cause any more damage. Take him to your doctor or to the hospital Accident and Emergency department. Make sure your child is up-to-date with his tetanus injections.

(I use magnesium sulphate paste for bringing infected spots 'to the boil' – it brings out any infection to the surface of the skin and then it just bursts in its own time. You can buy it from any chemist and you must cover the spot with a sticky plaster until *after it bursts*.)

STINGS

Children are often afraid of insects, even if they haven't been stung – perhaps because they look bigger to them than they do to us.

Bee, wasp and mosquito stings are more unpleasant than they are dangerous to children, UNLESS they are allergic to the sting, in which case they may develop anaphylactic shock, which can be very dangerous indeed (see 'Anaphylactic Shock' in Chapter 4 on Allergies and below).

WHAT TO DO

- For an ordinary insect sting, reassure and comfort the child. He will be frightened and in pain.

- Try and remove the sting, if there is one (wasps don't leave a sting). Hold a pair of tweezers as near to the skin as possible and pull it out quickly, as you would a stray eyebrow hair or a splinter. This may be difficult if the child is upset and struggling. If possible ask someone to hold him while you do this.

- DO NOT try to squeeze the sting out. It is contained in a poison sac and if you do squeeze it, you will force the poison into the skin and around the body.

- Put an ice-pack on the area around the sting. Bicarbonate of soda diluted with water (the amounts are written on the packet) will also help to relieve the pain and swelling.

- If the child seems ill after being stung, and you are worried, you must take him to the doctor (see 'Anaphylactic Shock' in Chapter 4 on Allergies and below).

If the child is stung in the mouth

He needs to go to hospital urgently. *The airway can swell up enough to stop the child breathing.*

(Don't let children drink fizzy drinks from cans – pour the drink into an open glass where insects can be seen. Wasps tend to crawl under the lid of the can and may be 'washed' out into the child's mouth when he takes a drink.)

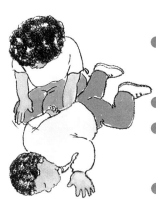

- Dial 999 to get an ambulance. Tell the operator what has happened. If the child is old enough, get him to suck on an ice cube, if not to take small sips of iced water.

- *Don't give anything to drink if the child starts to have difficulty breathing.*

- If your child is finding it difficult to breathe after an insect sting in the mouth, roll him quickly into the Recovery Position, keeping his airway as straight as you can.

- This child will probably be terrified. Soothe and reassure him as best you can by talking to him gently and calmly. Give him a favourite teddy to cuddle while he is lying down. Tell him what is happening and that you are waiting for the ambulance and are going with him to hospital.

- If he becomes unconscious, open his airway and keep an eye on his breathing. If it stops, start your ABC Resuscitation Routine right away.

> A for **AIRWAY**   (is it clear?)
>
> B for **BREATHING**   (is he breathing?)
>
> C for **CIRCULATION**   (is his heart beating?)

218

● If (to your knowledge) your child has not been stung before, *watch him very carefully* for the next few hours.

Anaphylactic shock

This is the name of a massive allergic reaction to an insect sting or an injection; it can also be caused by eating a food to which the child is allergic (see Chapter 4 on Allergies and Chapter 23 on Poisoning). It can develop after only a few seconds and is a medical emergency.

How to recognise this kind of reaction:

● A few seconds after the sting the child will develop all the signs of shock (see Chapter 27 on Shock).

REMEMBER – SHOCK LOOKS LIKE THIS

- ● His face may be very pale and grey-looking
- ● His skin may feel cold and clammy
- ● His pulse may feel fast and weak
- ● He may be frightened and fidgety
- ● He may be very thirsty
- ● He may yawn and 'gasp' for air
- ● He may say everything feels fuzzy
- ● He may become unconscious

● He may say he feels sick or may actually vomit.

● He may find it difficult to breathe, and may wheeze or gasp for air.

● He may have a sneezing attack.

● His face may start to swell up, particularly around the eyes and he may develop large red blotches on his skin, called urticaria.

● His pulse will be rapid and weak.

● The child may lose consciousness.

● THIS IS AN EMERGENCY. You must get the child to hospital as quickly as possible. Dial 999 to get an ambulance. Tell them exactly what has happened.

● Treat him for shock if he is still conscious. Talk to him calmly, tell him a doctor is coming, that you want him to lie down (this is the position that will help him most), and raise his legs on something like a cushion.

● If, however, he is having difficulty breathing, then you may sit him up, leaning forward with his arms on a table or cushions.

219

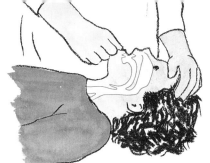

● If he becomes unconscious then quickly lie him down, open his airway and check his breathing. If it stops, start your ABC Resuscitation Routine until the ambulance arrives and you can get him to hospital (see Chapter 3 on ABC Resuscitation Routine).

> **A** for **AIRWAY**   (is it clear?)
>
> **B** for **BREATHING**   (is he breathing?)
>
> **C** for **CIRCULATION**   (is his heart beating?)

SWALLOWED SMALL OBJECTS

Children want to explore all the exciting and interesting things around them, and putting objects in their mouths and licking and sucking them is part of this process. They don't *mean* to swallow them but in the excitement of 'discovering' a new object, it may just slip down the throat – sometimes into the airway.

This is not naughtiness but part of a child's natural curiosity, and they must be taught NOT to put small things into their mouths which they *could* inhale or swallow. The other thing that may happen is that they are jogged or knocked when they are sucking something and they accidentally swallow it. Try to keep all small 'swallowable' objects out of the reach of small inquisitive fingers and mouths.

Coins and buttons are the common ones; these are unlikely to puncture or harm the gut, but the child could inhale them into the airway, where they can block it off. Sharp objects like pins or needles can do damage as they go down, whether it is to the food pipe (oesophagus), the stomach or the gut (see Chapter 2 on How the Body Works).

Batteries of any sort when swallowed, particularly the small hearing-aid or watch batteries, are *very dangerous* and need urgent hospital admission. They contain mercury and can kill a child. When you dial 999 for an ambulance, *tell the operator the child has swallowed a battery*.

KEEP ALL BATTERIES AWAY FROM SMALL CHILDREN.

Fish bones and chicken bones are swallowing favourites when older children try to eat too quickly. Make sure that when you give them this food most of the bones have been taken out or warn them that there are bones in the food. Quite often these bones may be swallowed with no ill effect. The child will then pass them out of his body in his stools.

WHAT TO DO

Fish and chicken bones may scratch on the way down.

- Try to encourage the child, if he is old enough, to have a piece of bread and a drink of water.

- If the child is unable to swallow, open his mouth and see if you can see the bone at the back of the throat. Fish bones, particularly if they are big, tend to get stuck in the tonsils. (Chicken bones tend to go lower down and can't easily be seen.)

- You may be able to reach the bone and gently pluck it out with a pair of tweezers. This needs a super-cool approach.

- Be very careful not to knock it further down the throat.

- If you are worried about your child take him to the doctor, or dial 999 for the ambulance.

- Whatever you do DON'T make the child 'sick the object up' – it might get stuck in the airway, which can do more harm than good.

(If the child *inhales* any of these objects, that is, breathes them into the air passages, rather than swallowing them into the stomach, follow Chapter 8 on Choking.)

TEETH

Babies are usually born without teeth (occasionally a new-born baby will have a tooth). Within three or four years children will have developed twenty 'milk' teeth. Once the child reaches about six years these teeth start to fall out, one by one, and he begins to get his adult teeth. There will eventually be thirty-two of these, all of which have to be looked after carefully for the rest of his life (see Chapter 2 on How the Body Works).

WHAT TO DO

A child may bleed from a tooth socket. This may be from a tooth that has been knocked out or has come out by itself. If it is an 'adult' tooth and it has been knocked out completely, there is a fair chance that the tooth could be re-implanted. If this happens to your child *try to find the tooth* – even if it has fallen in the mud, on a games pitch, for example.

It is important to wrap the tooth carefully in a clean tissue, or even better put it for safekeeping in a small amount of milk. Take the tooth to the dentist with the child as soon as you can. It is best to phone your dentist to warn him what has happened and to check that he can re-implant it.

221

If your dentist feels he can't help, either because of lack of experience or lack of time, try to get your child (and the tooth) to the local dental hospital where they probably will be able to do this delicate procedure. But time is important – the quicker the tooth can be put back the more successful it will be.

If it is a milk tooth don't worry – even if it wasn't wobbly, the new tooth will grow in its own time. Any bleeding will usually stop on its own, helped by cold water mouth-washes to which you can add a pinch of salt if the child will take it. The most important thing is to rinse around the tooth and wash the mouth out, to cut down the risk of infection.

If the bleeding doesn't stop (whether it is a milk or an adult tooth) ask the child to bite on a sterile or clean dressing – an eye-pad is ideal, (with the ties hanging outside the child's mouth so that there is no possibility of inhaling the pad). Keep the pressure up for about ten minutes. If it still does not stop by then, he should see a doctor.

Sit the child down quietly and encourage him to hold his head up and forward, letting the blood drain out. This position will help to stop the oozing.

DOG BITES

- Reassure and comfort the child – he will be terrified.
- Treat the child for shock.
- WASH and cover the wounds with a dry, clean cloth and bandage firmly enough to stop bleeding. Keep the limb raised.
- Get the child to a doctor as soon as you can.

FOR DEEP BITES

- Treat shock – he will almost certainly be shocked.
- Reassure and comfort him. Tell him what you are going to do.
- If you think he might be sick, roll him into the Recovery Position, keeping his airway open.
- DON'T let him touch any face wounds – you may have to stop him doing this by wrapping his arms in a blanket or towel.
- Call the ambulance by dialling 999. Tell them what has happened.

THINK

- Have you managed to get some help? Try shouting out of the window or front door.
- Have you called the ambulance? Try to get someone to do this for you.
- Have you checked for DANGER? (Have you got rid of the dog?)

IF YOUR CHILD IS BITTEN (OR LICKED) BY AN ANIMAL OUTSIDE THE UK there is a possibility that it could have rabies. If this happens to your child, this is what you do:

- Wash the area as soon as possible with clean (if possible), soapy water – or just water. If the child has been *bitten* (and not just licked), keep washing until you make the wound bleed.
- Immediately wash the wound with antiseptic.
- Cover the wounds with a dry, clean cloth.
- Keep the limb raised and *still*. Tie the legs together or tie the arm onto his chest, so that the infection does not move around the body.
- Then, *and not before*, get the child urgently to the medical treatment centre, for the special series of injections he needs.

SNAKE BITES

- Reassure and comfort the child. Treat him for shock.
- DON'T panic – most snake bites in the UK are NOT fatal.
- If possible, wash the bite mark thoroughly with warm, soapy water, cover with a dry, clean cloth and bandage in place.
- Keep the child as still as you can, so the poison doesn't get into the blood stream. *Lie him down* and then *keep the limb still* (tie one leg to the other or the arm to the chest).
- Call the ambulance by dialling 999. Tell them what has happened.
- If he is feeling sick, roll him into the Recovery Position.

THINK

- Have you called the ambulance? Try to get someone to do this for you.
- Have you checked for DANGER? (Have you got rid of the snake? REMEMBER to *get a description of the snake* before you do.)
- Shake and shout to the child to see if he is conscious.

IF THE CHILD BECOMES UNCONSCIOUS: be ready to start your ABC RESUSCITATION ROUTINE.

Now check 'A' for AIRWAY – is it clear?

IF HE DOESN'T RESPOND: OPEN THE AIRWAY. Tilt the child's head back and lift his chin forward. REMEMBER babies' necks are chubbier and more fragile. **Be gentle yet firm enough to tilt head back so airway is open.**

Now check 'B' for BREATHING

LOOK
LISTEN } for breathing
FEEL

IF THE CHILD IS NOT BREATHING: BREATHE FOR THE CHILD. Cover his mouth, or nose and mouth, with your mouth. Give him FIVE separate breaths. Watch his chest rise with each breath. *Less* breath for babies.

Now check 'C' for CIRCULATION

Is his heart beating? Feel the neck (or arm in a baby) for a pulse.

IF YOU CANNOT FEEL A PULSE: DO CHEST COMPRESSION. Feel for the right place – one finger-breadth below the nipple line. Press on the chest, at a rate of **100 presses per minute.**

For children over one year old: Use the 'heel' of one hand only, with your arm straight. **Press fifteen times to every two breaths** (so your hand presses in about 2.5-3.5cm or 1-1½ inches each time).

For babies: Use two fingers only and **press five times to one breath** (so your fingers press in about 2cm or about ¾ of an inch, each time).

KEEP DOING THIS UNTIL THE AMBULANCE ARRIVES.

STINGS (IN THE MOUTH) and ANAPHYLACTIC SHOCK

- Soothe and reassure the child. Tell him what is happening.
- Call for the ambulance by dialling 999. Tell them what has happened.
- DON'T give anything to drink if he is having difficulty breathing.
- His mouth and throat may start to swell up. If he is old enough, get him to suck on an ice-cube.
- If he is feeling sick or having trouble breathing, roll him quickly into the Recovery Position. Try to keep his airway open.

THINK

- Have you got help? Try shouting out of the window or front door.
- Have you called the ambulance? Try to get someone to do this for you.

IF THE CHILD BECOMES UNCONSCIOUS: be ready to start your ABC RESUSCITATION ROUTINE.

Now check 'A' for AIRWAY – is it clear?

IF HE DOESN'T RESPOND: OPEN THE AIRWAY. Tilt the child's head back and lift his chin forward. REMEMBER babies' necks are chubbier and more fragile. **Be gentle yet firm enough to tilt head back so airway is open.**

Now check 'B' for BREATHING

LOOK
LISTEN } for breathing
FEEL

IF THE CHILD IS NOT BREATHING: BREATHE FOR THE CHILD. Cover his mouth, or nose and mouth, with your mouth. Give him FIVE separate breaths. Watch his chest rise with each breath. *Less* breath for babies.

Now check 'C' for CIRCULATION

Is his heart beating? Feel the neck (or arm in a baby) for a pulse.

IF YOU CANNOT FEEL A PULSE: DO CHEST COMPRESSION. Feel for the right place – one finger-breadth below the nipple line. Press on the chest, at a rate of **100 presses per minute**.

For children over one year old: Use the 'heel' of one hand only, with your arm straight. **Press fifteen times to every two breaths** (so your hand presses in about 2.5-3.5cm or 1-1½ inches each time).

For babies: Use two fingers only and **press five times to one breath** (so your fingers press in about 2cm or about ¾ of an inch, each time).

KEEP DOING THIS UNTIL THE AMBULANCE ARRIVES.

23 POISONING

Over 2000 children receive hospital treatment each year having swallowed some sort of medicine or household product.

Poisons are substances that if taken into the body in a big enough dose can harm or kill a child. Most of the time poisoning is accidental but sometimes children playing around – with drugs or solvents, for instance – can take an overdose. Occasionally a child may deliberately play with solvents (see Chapter 14 on Drug Abuse, Solvent Sniffing and Alcohol) or want to kill herself (see Chapter 29 on Suicide).

Some substances that are poisonous to children are not poisonous to adults. Iron tablets can be lethal to children. So can alcohol. Children can become very ill and may even die after taking one measure of alcohol – especially if they decide to take a swig from the whisky or gin bottle. If you have the occasional swig please don't let the children see you do it! Try to keep all poisons in a place where they cannot be reached by children.

Children are curious and the younger ones especially like to explore everything with their mouths. They have no sense of danger and cannot be aware of what they are doing. So whether the child is sucking on a toy brick, which *can't* taste nice, or mummy's pills by the bed, which DO (they have a sugar coating), it doesn't really matter to her – but one of them can kill her, and one can't.

Poisons can get into the body in a variety of ways:

- *Through the mouth*, by eating or drinking something that is poisonous. (Remember: some plants in the garden if eaten or sucked can be poisonous, especially to children. If your child does this get her to hospital quickly and take the remains of the plant with you.)

- *Through the lungs*, by breathing in a variety of gases and fumes. These can be from fires, stoves, faulty appliances, chemicals (including solvents – some of which may be taken 'for fun'), or petrol engine exhausts.

- *By injection* into the skin, from a syringe (either accidentally or on purpose), or from a bite or sting from particular animals or reptiles, insects or even fish.

- *By being absorbed through the skin*, by contact with poisonous sprays and powders such as garden sprays, insecticides and some ordinary household substances – there are many of these which are particularly dangerous to a child, including white spirit, fire-lighters, bleach, some cosmetics, and of course rat poison. All of these should be KEPT OUT OF REACH OF CHILDREN.

All things that are poisonous to children are clearly marked on the bottle, jar or packet. You must always read the instructions. When it says POISON it means for adults and for children.

What can happen when a child is poisoned?

Once in the body, poisons can act in a variety of ways:

These are the symbols to warn you of danger.

- Some act on the central nervous system and may poison the brain, in which case the child may quickly lose consciousness, or stop breathing, or her heart may stop.

- Some act by poisoning the muscles, preventing them from working properly, and in some cases would make the heart (the most important muscle) stop altogether.

- Some act by preventing the exchange of gases (oxygen and carbon dioxide) in the lungs and the child's breathing will then be affected.

- Some act directly on the child's food passages causing her to vomit, have diarrhoea and terrible tummy ache. *Any severe vomiting and diarrhoea in a child is an emergency and she should be seen by a doctor as quickly as possible* (see Chapter 12 on Diarrhoea and Vomiting).

- Some poisons are corrosive and may severely burn the child's lips, mouth, gullet and stomach, causing a great deal of pain, injury and distress.

WHAT TO LOOK FOR

- She may tell you she has taken something she shouldn't have.

- She may look weird or 'not herself' (if she is not showing obvious signs that she has been poisoned).

- She may show you, or you may find, a container near where she was playing.

- You may see scalds and burns on her lips or around her mouth.

- An older child, whom you suspect of glue-sniffing, may develop an odd smell about her, or she may be behaving in a way that is just not her – either very 'down' or unusually noisy and giggly. She may seem as if she is drunk (see Chapter 14 on Drug Abuse, Solvent Sniffing and Alcohol).

WHAT TO DO

- If possible, ask her what has happened, if she has swallowed anything that mummy didn't give her and if so, WHAT?

227

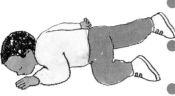

● DO NOT in any circumstances, make the child vomit – it could make the situation worse.

● If she is becoming unconscious, put her in the Recovery Position, to prevent her inhaling any vomit.

● Be aware that her airway could become blocked, particularly if she starts to fit (see Chapter 17 on Fits).

● Be prepared to start your ABC Resuscitation Routine if necessary.

> **A** for **AIRWAY** (is it clear?)
>
> **B** for **BREATHING** (is she breathing?)
>
> **C** for **CIRCULATION** (is her heart beating?)

● If your child stops breathing and has swallowed something caustic – you can usually tell because there will be burns around the area of the mouth – try not to burn your mouth by putting it onto her mouth. You won't be able to think or act clearly if you are in pain yourself.

Wipe away as much of the poison as possible. Put a handkerchief or tissue over her mouth and try to breathe through this for protection.

REMEMBER: *Poisons act more quickly on children, with much more dramatic and sometimes devastating effects.*

DO NOT GIVE HER ANYTHING TO EAT OR DRINK even if you feel it would neutralise the poison. It won't, and it will only make a bad situation worse.

GET MEDICAL HELP QUICKLY – tell them what has happened, and particularly, if you know, what the child has been poisoned with.

If it is possible, *take any bottles or containers with you to the hospital* so that the substance the child has swallowed or injected can be analysed immediately (see Chapter 14 on Drug Abuse, Solvent Sniffing and Alcohol).

- Reassure and comfort the child.
- DO NOT make the child sick – this may make matters worse.
- DO NOT give her anything to eat or drink.
- If the child feels sick, roll her over into the Recovery Position.
- Call the ambulance by dialling 999. Tell them what has happened.
- Take any bottle or container with you to hospital.

THINK

- Have you managed to get some help? Try shouting out of the window or front door.
- Have you called the ambulance? Try to get someone to do this for you.
- Have you checked for DANGER?
- Shake and shout to the child to see if she is conscious.

IF THE CHILD BECOMES UNCONSCIOUS: be ready to start your ABC RESUSCITATION ROUTINE.

Now check 'A' for AIRWAY – is it clear?

IF SHE DOESN'T RESPOND: OPEN THE AIRWAY. Tilt the child's head back and lift her chin forward. REMEMBER babies' necks are chubbier and more fragile. **Be gentle yet firm enough to tilt head back so airway is open.**

Now check 'B' for BREATHING

LOOK
LISTEN } for breathing
FEEL

IF THE CHILD IS NOT BREATHING: BREATHE FOR THE CHILD. Cover her mouth, or nose and mouth, with your mouth. Give her FIVE separate breaths. Watch her chest rise with each breath. REMEMBER you need *less* breath for babies.

Now check 'C' for CIRCULATION

Is her heart beating? Check for the pulse. Feel the neck (or arm in a baby) for a pulse. **If there is no pulse and you haven't got help GET IT NOW.**

IF YOU CANNOT FEEL A PULSE: DO CHEST COMPRESSION. Feel for the right place – one finger-breadth below the nipple line. Press on the chest, at a rate of **100 presses per minute.**

For children over one year old: Use the 'heel' of one hand only, with your arm straight. **Press fifteen times to every two breaths** (so your hand presses in about 2.5-3.5cm or 1-1½ inches each time).

For babies: Use two fingers only and **press five times to one breath** (so your fingers press in about 2cm which is about ¾ of an inch, each time).

KEEP DOING THIS UNTIL THE AMBULANCE ARRIVES.

24 PREGNANCY IN ADOLESCENCE

Girls need to know early on about their periods, so that when they begin – remember this can be as early as eight or nine years old – it doesn't come as too much of a shock. (Boys should be told too so that they can understand from quite a young age why girls get grumpy sometimes for no apparent good reason!) Girls and boys should both realise that once a girl's periods start, she could get pregnant after sexual intercourse.

Adolescent girls who have unprotected sex run a high risk of pregnancy because that is when they are most fertile. They may have been forced to have sex against their will, or have sexual feelings that they cannot or don't want to control. Sometimes teenage girls have sex because it is another way, possibly the only way, that they can get cuddles and affection.

There is no easy answer when a teenager becomes pregnant, because whatever way she chooses to deal with it, it may affect her for the rest of her life.

Parents must be aware that this could happen. Childline counsellors receive many calls from girls who are terrified to tell their parents they are pregnant – and some from children who have been slung out of the family home because of it. One way to avoid this is to give children (and this includes boys) as much information as early as possible, so they know as much as they can when their hormones take over. Some parents find this difficult to do.

It is important for parents to recognise that *their* teenager is as likely to be having sex as any other teenager. That sounds pretty obvious but we, as parents, all tend not to recognise what is happening even when it is staring us in the face.

The message to teenagers must be that, 'We don't want to encourage you to have sex but, if you do, tell us *early on* because the earlier you tell us the more options there are available.' For instance, emergency contraception works up to seventy-two hours after intercourse. It is taken in two doses, twelve hours apart. It is available on prescription from your doctor or from the local family planning clinic.

There is another new pill called RU486 which, if taken within *sixty-three* days after having sexual intercourse, will abort (get rid of) the foetus. The girl will feel a certain amount of discomfort – maybe even pain, rather like a period pain – as the lining of the womb comes away and with it the pregnancy.

It is important that teenagers have enough information to know how to recognise if they are pregnant – in other words, they miss a period, they may feel sick and their breasts may swell up. Try to make sure that your daughter would feel able to tell you if she has had un-protected sex.

You should find out whether the local health authority runs a family planning clinic for young people, particularly if your daughter is under sixteen years old. (It is now within the law for contraceptives to be pre-scribed to an under-sixteen-year-old, as long as the doctor feels that she is aware of what she is doing.) You need to make sure that your teen-agers are aware of it; where it is and what it does – that is, provides contraception (and referral for abortion) to teenagers *without their own doctor knowing anything about it – if they don't want him to – and without you knowing either!*

It is quite a good idea to put the name and address of the family planning clinic up on the notice board, or stick it on the kitchen wall, along with the local Brook Advisory Service number. This will save them the agonising decision of having to tell you and they may be en-couraged to get help more quickly if they get into any kind of trouble.

Safe Sex

Parents (and children) really have not yet got to grips with the AIDS situation. It is a real threat to young life and awful though it is, the whole issue has to be faced more honestly.

Young people must use condoms *as well as* taking or using any other method of contraception. Condoms are the only sure way to cut down the risk of being infected with the AIDS virus and other sexually trans-mitted diseases, although they may not be the chosen way to avoid the girl getting pregnant. Obviously the more partners teenagers have, the more at risk they are of getting AIDS or any of the other diseases they can catch from having sex.

All of these things need courage if you are a parent. Courage to recognise the dangers, courage to give the right information to help teenagers make sensible *informed* choices, and courage to help them get it right – like putting up the information in a place where they can get to it, and even putting a box of condoms in the bathroom drawer and replacing it when it is empty (without asking any questions).

One way to make sure that your teenagers know as much as possible about sex education (apart from school – where, in any case, they prob-ably learn more from their mates than they do from the teachers) is to buy them some really good books – ones which grip them from the moment they open the page and give them bags of information that *they really want to know.* You can leave the books lying around if you don't feel like talking to them directly. Some parents find it easier than others to talk to their children about sex – the secret is to start early in their lives so it doesn't become such a big deal when it really matters.

231

If your daughter (or son), or a child you know, doesn't want to see her own doctor about anything to do with her sexuality, she needn't. She has a choice of going to her nearest family planning clinic, or to one a friend has recommended. It is a *self-referral* system which means that the consumer – in this case the young person – can choose.

As far as an unwanted pregnancy is concerned, abortion (by operation, rather than taking a pill) is one of the options. However, doctors are understandably reluctant to give an under-sixteen-year-old a general anaesthetic without parental consent. She will have to be seen by a doctor – either at the local family planning clinic, her own GP, or ideally at the Brook Advisory Centre (ideally, because they are geared up to the problems of young people). Any of these doctors will help the *girl in confidence* to come to the best decision as to what to do about the pregnancy. None of the solutions is easy.

Abortion is not without its downside. Teenagers must be counselled beforehand. It is really important to understand what a devastating effect abortion can have on some young women – there are some who feel that there is no other experience that has affected their lives so much, even years after the event. However, some women just feel overwhelming relief at no longer having an unwanted pregnancy.

Sometimes a young woman may feel she has no one to turn to and may try to deal with the situation herself, or she could miscarry – she may not even have realised that she was pregnant. Fortunately, today there is no need for anyone to feel so alone. The 'Brook' is well used to dealing sympathetically, honestly and confidentially with all teenagers' problems. They won't be fazed by anything they are told and the service is free.

If your child has an extremely heavy period particularly if she is in a lot of pain, *she may have miscarried*. You must ensure that she sees a doctor; *it needn't be her GP*. It can be the local family planning clinic – they can make an NHS referral to see a gynaecologist (a doctor who specialises in women's – even very young women's – problems). Alternatively, the Brook Advisory Centres will also see her (and you, if she wants that) and refer her on to a doctor who will be able to help. Both of these services are in absolute confidence.

If your daughter is sexually active or she has been sexually abused or raped (see Chapter 26 on Sexual Abuse) and you feel that there is a chance she could become pregnant or is at risk in some other way, she or you may want to contact:

The Brook Advisory Centres
Central Office, 153A East Street, London SE17 2SD.
Tel. 071 708 1234/1390 (for referral to your local centre)

Brook Advisory Centres provide free, confidential birth control advice and supplies, and help with emotional or sexual problems. They have also published an excellent guide for teenagers called *Say Yes, Say No, Say Maybe* by Susie Hayman.

Marie Stopes Clinic
Well Woman Centre, 108 Whitfield Street, London W1P 6BE.
Tel. 071 388 0662

Margaret Pyke Centre
15 Bateman Buildings, Soho Square, London W1V 5TW.
Tel. 071 734 9351

Rape Crisis Centre
PO Box 69, London WC1X 9NJ.
Twenty-four-hour telephone service: 071 837 1600

Look in the telephone directory for details of these centres in your area.

If your child or a child you know is troubled in this (or any other way) she might like to phone **Childline**. This is a twenty-four-hour confidential counselling service.

Childline Freefone: 0800 1111

OR your child might like to *write* to:

Childline
Freepost 1111, London N1 0BR.

The Family Planning Association run a mail order bookshop called Healthwise. They will gladly give parents any information to help them cope with teenage sexuality. Healthwise staff are helpful, knowledgeable and sensitive to these issues. They will give advice over the phone about the many books they have in stock, or you can get a catalogue by sending them a stamped addressed envelope.

Healthwise
Family Planning Association, 27-35 Mortimer Street, London W1N 7RJ.
Tel. 071 636 7866

You may find the following books interesting and helpful: *Have You Started Yet?* by Ruth Thomson (Pan); *It's OK to be You: Feeling Good about Growing Up* by Claire Patterson and Lindsay Quilter (Piccolo); and *Making it from 12 to 20 – How to Survive Your Teens* by Alexandra and Iain Parsons (Judy Piatkus Publishers Ltd).

233

25 RABIES

This is a particularly unpleasant and fatal disease which affects dogs and some other animals. They can pass it to each other and to humans by 'injecting' their saliva into the body when they bite. Humans have less than a one-in-four chance of catching rabies after being bitten, scratched or licked by a 'rabid' animal. But if they do catch rabies and are not treated they will die. There is no known cure once it takes hold of the body.

Rabies was present in Britain in the last century, but due to the law which forbids dogs and other animals to enter the country unless they are in quarantine for six months (while they are carefully watched for signs of the disease), it has died out.

In the early 1980s it looked as if rabies was going to make a spectacular – and worrying – comeback into Britain, but the experts now think this is unlikely. This is mostly because of the Wildlife Vaccination Programme which has controlled the disease but not got rid of it completely.

However, rabies is very common in some countries where dogs are allowed to run wild. This happens particularly in India, but some countries in Europe (including France) have many animals with rabies.

If you are travelling abroad the child must NEVER stroke or touch any animal – *even* a dog or cat. Even if the child is only licked by a rabid animal she can be infected through the smallest scratch or cut on her skin, because the disease is carried in the animal's saliva (spit). This is extremely serious and usually fatal if the child is not treated quickly.

If a dog or cat bites or licks your child in a foreign country and the animal is not known to you or you think it might have rabies you must get medical help URGENTLY. There is an injection that can be given to treat your child which will counteract the disease that the animal might have been carrying.

WHAT TO DO

- As soon as the child is bitten WASH THE AREA straightaway with plenty of clean, if possible soapy, water. Keep washing it until you make the wound bleed. Obviously, if the child is only licked you don't make it bleed. The important thing is to wash the germs off the skin.

- If possible, immediately flush out the wound with an antiseptic.

ONLY AFTER WASHING THE WOUND IN THIS WAY SHOULD YOU THEN GET THE CHILD TO THE URGENT SPECIALISED MEDICAL HELP SHE NEEDS.

- If there are any deep fang wounds, cover them with a clean, dry dressing until she sees the doctor. Keep the limb raised, if possible, to control any bleeding.

- You need to get her to where she can get a rabies ('post-exposure') vaccine urgently. The sooner she has prompt medical treatment with the proper vaccine the better are her chances of recovery. This will probably be at one of the special treatment centres that are set up in many countries in the Developing World to deal with this problem. If there isn't one near you, get her to a hospital. If they cannot help her, they will tell you the best place to go.

- The child will then be given the rabies vaccine, which is a daily course of injections. Make sure you ask for the new MODERN VACCINE. The 'old' one can have extremely nasty side-effects; but if this is all that is available at the treatment centre you go to, then have the first injection there – the sooner the child is treated the better – and then ask where you can go to get the modern vaccine.

It is unlikely that your child will be bitten by a rabid animal. However, we do occasionally see rabies in the UK and it gets into the country because people think that it 'wouldn't harm' just to take the family dog or cat along with them in the car when they go for their short break across the Channel or wherever. Perhaps they couldn't find anyone to look after their pet whilst they were away and genuinely couldn't see the harm of doing this. If their pet then encounters another dog or cat, or a wild animal such as a fox, and that animal is rabid, chances are . . . It is just not worth taking the risk. Rabies is a killer.

Alternatively, children are suckers for animals in cages. Abroad, they may see some poor animal cooped up and manage to persuade their unsuspecting parent to take it home. The animal may be rabid.

If you are travelling with the children for a long period, or even just on holiday, to places where rabies is not controlled, you may want to consider having the new rabies vaccine *before you go*. Your GP will have information about this.

Please REMEMBER wherever you are abroad to keep your children away from all stray animals, no matter how friendly they are. Remember they will rarely attack unless they are provoked. In this instance 'provoked' can be as simple as being stroked.

- Reassure and comfort the child – she will be terrified.
- Treat the child for shock.
- WASH the area as soon as possible with clean (if possible), soapy water – or just water. If the child has been *bitten* and not just licked, keep washing the wound until you make it bleed.
- IMMEDIATELY wash the wound (and the skin around the wound) with antiseptic.
- Cover the wounds with a clean, dry cloth.
- Keep the limb raised and *still*. Tie the child's legs together or tie her arm to her chest, so that the poison does not move around the body.
- Then *and not before* get the child to a medical treatment centre URGENTLY for the special series of injections that she needs.

SEXUAL ABUSE

26

No matter how difficult sexual abuse is for most of us even to think about, some children, often very young ones, are being abused in this way. This means that they are being made to have sex *against their will* or are being made to take part in sexual acts with people they may, or may not, know.

It is important for parents and carers to get to grips with sexual abuse because pretending it doesn't happen will not stop it happening.

So as not to confuse, in this chapter I have called the child 'she' and the abuser 'he'. I know this may not always be the case as *boys are sexually abused as much as girls*. Parents must know how best to protect their children and how to recognise any worrying signs that will alert them to the fact that something may be wrong.

Parents have to be sensible, watchful and clear-thinking without worrying unnecessarily. There is no reason on earth why normal, loving families should feel they can't cuddle and comfort each other, just as they have always done. However, if by any chance a child describes things that have been happening to her, then no matter how unbelievable they may seem you must listen. Children don't tend to make up this sort of thing – the words are just not in their everyday vocabulary.

One of the most worrying things for parents to cope with is that most children who are being sexually abused *know* their abuser. BUT they may not have known him for very long.

Abused children may be 'targeted', which means that the abuser picks a child he fancies and weaves a web that takes patience and cunning. These people will stop at nothing to move the chosen child into their fantasy.

One of the things that sometimes happens is this. The abuser befriends the parents over quite a long period, maybe six months, and then, when the parents trust him, he invites the child to go out fishing or on a picnic – some event that is a great treat. No abuse may take place until after the umpteenth outing and then it starts – the abuser knows he's safe. Who's going to believe the child now?

This is not a 'one-off' incident. The police department dealing with these cases say abusers have a whole 'courting' ritual that they use over and over again and parents should be aware of it.

If the abuser is known to the child – he may even be a family friend or relative – then the child may be afraid of telling a parent. This may be for a variety of reasons. The child may think that she wouldn't be believed, the abuser may have threatened to hurt her (or hurt her parents, brothers or sisters) if she says anything; she may think that by telling she would split up the family. (This also applies to boys.)

Alternatively, if the child has been abused from an early age, she may not even realise that what she is being expected to do is not normal.

WHAT TO LOOK FOR

- Your child may start acting in a way you don't recognise, such as becoming very secretive – or very aggressive.

- She may start wetting the bed.

- She may appear restless and be unable to sit still or she may have un-explained temper tantrums.

- She may refuse to go to school.

- She may do none of these things – but she just seems 'different'.

- The child may be very distressed.

- The child might bleed from her vagina. If your child is *not* coming up to puberty – and remember some girls start their periods as young as eight years old – it could mean that she has been sexually abused.

- The child might bleed from the anus.

THERE MAY BE NO BLEEDING FROM THE ANUS OR THE VAGINA IN CHILD SEXUAL ABUSE.

- If you suspect sexual abuse, there may also be other signs. There may be redness or itching, bruising, soreness or even tears in and around the vagina or anus. Or there may be none of these things.

- You might see some bruises or marks on your child's body that may worry you – there may also be what look like burns.

  If you see unexplained bites, burns or other marks either on your child or a child you are looking after, you should tell someone about them.

  If you are the parent, talk to your child about how she thinks she got the 'marks' on her body. Don't say immediately that you recognise them – they may not be what you think anyway. She may be pleased to talk about them and there may be some simple explanation, or she may find it difficult to tell you, in which case try not to push her. She may not be ready to talk to you but make sure she realises that you are ready to listen to her whenever she wants.

  You might want to go and talk to the teacher in case the child is being bullied, or you might find it easier to go and talk to your Health Visitor or doctor.

  If you are a teacher or carer you might start by telling the parents about the marks and that you are concerned. However, if you continue to see them and if you feel for some reason the parent is not taking the situation seriously enough, then call your local doctor or have a chat with the Health Visitor.

There may be some simple explanation, or it may be that the child is being bullied. There is also the possibility that the child is being abused in some way.

- If you feel your child could have been a victim of sexual abuse, you might gently ask her if she would like you to look at her bottom. If you are her father, however, and you feel uncomfortable about doing this, perhaps you might prefer to ask a female member of the family to do this for you – it may depend on the age of the child and how urgent the situation is.

- Don't hesitate to contact your GP or Health Visitor right away – they are trained to deal with these sorts of situations and, if it is happening, they will know how to help you and your child.

WHAT TO DO

- Try to comfort and reassure your child. If she or he has been sexually abused, the child will be terrified and very distressed.

- If you notice any of the things discussed *in someone else's child* you obviously have to tread even more carefully. DON'T attempt to examine the child's bottom yourself in any circumstances. If it is possible, mention your worries to the parent. It takes guts to do this and you will have to pick your moment and handle it sensitively. (Just imagine if it were your child and someone had *possibly* got it wrong.) You may feel that you could only do this through a trusted third person – perhaps another member or close friend of the family – perhaps even the teacher at school.

- If the situation continues to worry you and you feel that there is a risk that the child is being abused, then you may want to talk in confidence to your local GP or Health Visitor. However, these people may not be right for you – you may not have a good enough relationship with them to make you feel you can talk openly about this problem. You might, therefore, like to approach the NSPCC. This organisation is staffed by trained social workers who are extremely sympathetic to the problems people have in recognising and *dealing with* a child who is being sexually abused. Or you could go to your local Social Services Department (address in telephone directory). Social workers are bound *by law* to help in any way they can with a child who may be being badly treated in any way.

Always be aware, however, that 'media hype' – over-reaction in newspapers and television – would have us believe that every other child is the victim of sexual abuse. It IS a very worrying problem and one which parents must constantly be on their guard against. However, it is all too easy to jump to the wrong conclusions, particularly in someone else's child.

Organisations that can help

If you are worried in any way that a child you know might be sexually abused or being hurt or abused in any other way, you may want to talk about it to someone.

If you feel that *you* are out of control with the feelings that you have towards your child or children (by being violent or ill-treating them in some way) you may want to talk about it to someone, and you may need help.

If you think that your child might be sexually abused or generally ill-treated *within your family* and you don't feel in control of the situation, or you are finding it difficult to face up to what is happening, it might help to talk to someone who will listen and will understand what you are going through.

In any of these situations, you might like to contact a new organisation set up by the NSPCC, called the NSPCC Child Protection Helpline. It is a twenty-four-hour *confidential* counselling service, run by qualified social workers for anyone who might want to get help or ask advice about child sexual abuse. (Confidential means that no one else need know about your problems, unless you want that to happen.) The Freefone telephone number is:

NSPCC Child Protection Helpline 0800 800 500

Remember 0800 (freefone) numbers do not show on itemised telephone bills.

The NSPCC also have a helpful leaflet for parents and carers called *Protect Your Child*. You can send for it by writing to:

NSPCC
67 Saffron Hill, London EC1N 8RS.

If you feel that a troubled child you know might like to talk to someone *in total confidence* on the telephone, he or she should ring Childline. This is a free twenty-four-hour confidential service. The switchboard operator will transfer the child to a trained counsellor. It is sometimes difficult to get through to Childline because so many children ring in, but she *will* get through eventually. The Freefone telephone number is:

Childline 0800 1111

OR the child might like to write in confidence to Childline. The address (no stamp needed) is:

Childline, Freepost 1111, London N1 0BR.

If as a parent, you have problems that you feel would be helped by talking, either to other parents or to an organisation set up to listen to parents' problems, you might like to contact Parentline which is run by parents for parents. This is a twenty-four-hour service (after 5 p.m. there is an answerphone which will tell you the number of a volunteer you can speak to). There are twenty-five branches throughout the country. If there isn't one in your town you can ring this central number for your nearest branch. Their telephone number is:

Parentline 0268 757077

Parents Anonymous provide 'a sympathetic ear'. They stress they are *not* trained counsellors but will listen to problems and point parents in the direction of local organisations that will be able to give specific help and support.

Their telephone number is:

Parents Anonymous 071 263 8918

If you would like to read more about the issue of child abuse and keeping your child safe, there are several books available: *Keeping Safe* (Hodder & Stoughton) and *The Willow Street Kids* (Pan/Piccolo) both by Michele Elliott, Director of Kidscape; and *We Can Say No!* by David Pithers and Sarah Green (Arrow).

27 SHOCK

Shock is one of those terms that is bandied about but no one quite knows what it is. Basically it means a dropping-off of the blood supply to the most important organs in the body – the heart, lungs and brain.

When a child goes 'into shock', she will usually have had some sort of accident, where she has lost fluid such as blood or is in a lot of pain. It can even occur following very severe diarrhoea.

A child left in shock can die unless she is given the right treatment quickly.

When a child is in shock, her body drains a lot of the blood away from the parts that don't need it – like the skin, hands and feet – and takes it straight to the parts that do, such as the brain, heart, lungs and kidneys.

Unfortunately this doesn't always happen and this is where the danger lies. These organs to which the blood is being sent may start to act in a peculiar way. The child's blood pressure may drop and she may stop passing urine. She may lose consciousness.

WHAT TO LOOK FOR

This is what a child with shock may look like:

- *Her face may be very pale and grey-looking.* Her lips may look blue, and the inside of her lips will look pale and drained of blood.

- *Her skin may feel cold and clammy.* You may see beads of sweat on her top lip.

- *Her pulse may feel fast and weak* because the heart has to work harder, but there is less blood to pump around the body (in bleeding and burns).

- *The child may feel frightened and fidgety*; an older child may be unusually talkative.

- *She may say she is thirsty.* This is the body's natural urge to put back the fluid that has been lost. But you must NOT give her a drink.

- *She may yawn or 'gasp' for air.* This also is a natural bodily response to try to replace the oxygen lost in the blood.

- *She may tell you that everything feels 'fuzzy'* or she may not seem to know where she is or what has happened to her. If she is standing up, she may faint. She may look 'odd'. This is the brain's response to a low blood supply.

242

- *She may become unconscious.*

CAUSES OF SHOCK

- *Bleeding*. When a child loses blood the problem has to be tackled quickly. Children's bodies react more seriously and more dramatically to injury than adults' bodies (see Chapter 6 on Bleeding).

- *Burns* cause large volumes of fluid 'serum' (straw-coloured liquid) to leak out of the burnt areas of skin (see Chapter 7 on Burns and Scalds).

- *Diarrhoea and vomiting* can have disastrous effects on a small child, and even worse on a baby. They cannot cope with the sudden violent loss of fluid.

- *Severe pain* from injury after an accident, for example, or appendicitis. (Alternatively, she may be in shock without a lot of pain, and you will have less of a clue to what is the matter – see 'Internal bleeding' in Chapter 6 on Bleeding.)

- *Sweating* caused by a very high temperature. (This doesn't happen in babies.)

WHAT TO DO

- Send for medical help as quickly as you can (especially if your child is badly injured). Ring for an ambulance by dialling 999 and explain why you are calling. Or if possible get someone else to do it for you.

- Do NOT give her anything to eat or drink, even if she tells you she is thirsty, although you can wipe her lips with a clean, wet hanky or face-cloth.

- Talk calmly and sensibly to your child. Tell her what you are doing even though you may think she cannot hear you or is too badly injured to take any notice. Shock is made worse by anxiety or panic, and if she can hear your voice she will realise you are there and it will reassure her.

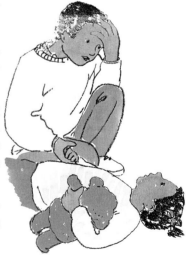

- Put her in the Recovery Position if you think she might be sick, otherwise just make her comfortable. If she is lying on a cold surface, put a blanket or a coat underneath her and cover her with a light blanket. Roll her gently to place the blanket under her body.

- Treat her injuries or deal with her illness as best you can while you are waiting for a doctor or for the ambulance to arrive.

- Keep her as still as possible. If she is in a bad state of shock she may be very restless. Try to calm her with your voice and try to distract her, perhaps by reading her a story, by remembering some very happy event, or by thinking of something exciting that is going to happen in the near future. (Don't worry too much about the possibility that she

243

may NOT be able to go. If she is that ill or badly injured, she won't be aware of time and it may take her mind off her situation for a little while.)

● If her lower limbs are not broken it may help to raise her legs.

● Keep her warm and comfortable. DO NOT make her too hot. This would take the blood away from the parts of the body that really need it, such as the heart and lungs. DO NOT use electric blankets, hot-water bottles or heaps of blankets, no matter how shivery she feels.

● WATCH HER CAREFULLY. If she becomes unconscious, ask yourself, is she safe? Open her airway and check her breathing. If it stops, you must start your ABC Resuscitation Routine.

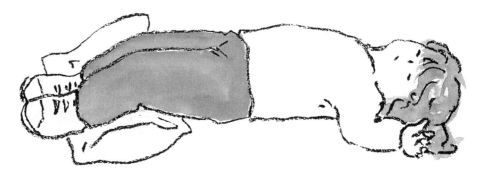

A for **AIRWAY** (is it clear?)

B for **BREATHING** (is she breathing?)

C for **CIRCULATION** (is her heart beating?)

Once she gets to hospital

They may possibly put up a 'drip' to help put back the amount of fluid she has lost. (If she is in a bad state of shock and there is a Paramedic in the ambulance, this may be started BEFORE she gets to hospital.) The fluid is given through a small needle in the vein and it literally drips into the body. If she has lost a lot of blood she may be given plasma – the straw-coloured liquid part of blood – until such time as she is 'cross-matched' (blood that is tested to find the right type and Rhesus-factor for your child) and then she will be given blood. All blood is AIDS-tested to make it as safe as possible for transfusion. The ambulance crew may also give her oxygen through a face mask if they think she needs it.

The doctor may give her pain-killers if she needs them, either by mouth or by injection into the muscle or vein. Occasionally they give drugs by a suppository which is placed in the anus (back-passage). If

244

she has a 'drip', particularly if she is unconscious, any drugs will probably be put into the drip bottle and given to her through the vein – which is the quickest way of getting drugs into the body.

If she has any infection it will be treated with antibiotics.

If she has to have an operation she will be taken to the operating theatre. Sometimes, if she is very dehydrated (dangerously lacking in fluid) the doctor will wait to operate until the fluid in her body has been safely replaced by the 'drip'. When her body has taken back all the fluid that is needed, it is safe enough for her to have an anaesthetic.

The medical staff will ask you if she has eaten or drunk anything recently. It is dangerous for a child to have an anaesthetic with anything in her tummy – she might be sick and inhale the vomit. If it is an emergency and she has eaten recently they may have to pass a tube into the stomach to empty it out. This is unpleasant but absolutely necessary if she needs emergency surgery.

Ask if you can stay with her (if you want to) during any emergency procedures the medical team have to do (see 'Taking a Child to Hospital' in Chapter 1 on Preparation and Practical Issues).

- Reassure and comfort the child. Tell her what you are going to do.
- Loosen her clothes at the neck and chest.
- Roll her gently into the Recovery Position.
- Ring for the ambulance by dialling 999. Tell them what has happened.

THINK

- Have you managed to get some help? Try shouting out of the window or front door.
- Have you called the ambulance? Try to get someone to do this for you.
- Have you checked for DANGER?

IF THE CHILD BECOMES UNCONSCIOUS: be ready to start your ABC RESUSCITATION ROUTINE.

Now check   'A' for AIRWAY – is it clear?

IF SHE DOESN'T RESPOND: OPEN THE AIRWAY. Tilt the child's head back and lift her chin forward. REMEMBER babies' necks are chubbier and more fragile. **Be gentle yet firm enough to tilt head back so airway is open.**

Now check   'B' for BREATHING

LOOK
LISTEN } for breathing
FEEL

IF THE CHILD IS NOT BREATHING: BREATHE FOR THE CHILD. Cover her mouth, or nose and mouth, with your mouth. Give her FIVE separate breaths. Watch her chest rise with each breath. REMEMBER you need *less* breath for babies.

Now check   'C' for CIRCULATION

Is her heart beating? Check for the pulse. Feel the neck (or arm in a baby) for a pulse. **If there is no pulse and you haven't got help GET IT NOW.**

IF YOU CANNOT FEEL A PULSE: DO CHEST COMPRESSION. Feel for the right place – one finger-breadth below the nipple line. Press on the chest, at a rate of **100 presses per minute**.

For children over one year old: Use the 'heel' of one hand only, with your arm straight. **Press fifteen times to every two breaths** (so your hand presses in about 2.5-3.5cm or 1-1½ inches each time).

For babies: Use two fingers only and **press five times to one breath** (so your fingers press in about 2cm which is about ¾ of an inch, each time).

KEEP DOING THIS UNTIL THE AMBULANCE ARRIVES.

SUFFOCATION

Children suffocate when they are not able to get enough air into their lungs because of something blocking their airway *from the outside* (rather than something which they have inhaled, for instance). There are many things that can cause a child to suffocate: these include plastic bags, soft pillows, or sand – if their heads are covered accidentally or even on purpose on the beach or in the sand pit. A child can also suffocate from inhaling smoke from a fire.

PLASTIC BAGS

Keep plastic bags (and all forms of plastic packaging and wrapping – such as cling film) AWAY FROM CHILDREN. For some reason children love them, the way they feel, the way they mould and crackle perhaps . . . But why they want to put them over their heads is a mystery. However, enough children have died in this way to convince us that, whatever the reason, plastic bags *are* a dangerous attraction and parents need to be aware of this.

What happens is this. As soon as the bag goes over the child's face and the child breathes in, the bag clings to the face and the child will be *unable to remove the bag*. As he panics so he breathes in again but *there is no air left in the bag to breathe* – this whole process only takes seconds. The child will die if the bag isn't removed quickly – by tearing or cutting a hole in it to let the air in and release the pressure. The child, particularly a little one, will probably not be able to remove the bag himself after the first breath.

One of the tragedies of children sniffing solvents is that sometimes they use plastic bags to concentrate the fumes and the child can suffocate by accident while he is sniffing. (See Chapter 14 on Drug Abuse, Solvent Sniffing and Alcohol.)

SAND

Sand pits and beaches are great favourites with children and are usually the safest places for them to play *as long as they are supervised*. Occasionally, however, accidents happen. There is a game children play where they cover each other with sand, so much so that they can't even wiggle their toes. If they do, the sand 'cover' collapses and everyone falls about laughing. Great fun, except if a child gets too carried away and covers another child's *face*. (How could a small child understand that this is dangerous?)

Another possibility is that the child might get caught in a fall of sand or earth, for instance on a building site, or when he is playing in a big mound of sand conveniently dumped in your road or driveway by your local council or the builder.

SOFT PILLOWS

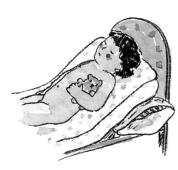

Children under one year old should not have pillows – and I wouldn't rush to give them one even when they are over a year old. If and when you do, it is better that the pillow is firm, not too fat and made of a man-made fibre (not one made from feathers or down) so that you can bung it in the washing machine when you need to.

If the child has a cold and is snuffly, he is probably better propped up, but put the pillow underneath the head end of the mattress, not directly underneath the child. (See 'Coughs and Colds' in Chapter 22 on Minor Injuries and Illnesses.)

DON'T use 'squashy' make-shift pillows.

Baby nests, duvets and cot bumpers: Make sure these are approved by BSI (British Standards Institute) – their 'kite' mark will be on the product – to keep your child safe.

SHEEPSKINS

Don't use these for babies and toddlers. They get too hot and can easily suffocate in the long hairs.

BEAN BAGS

Keep babies and toddlers away from these. They are great for older kids to bounce on, or the dog to sleep on, but they are *dangerous* for little ones who may get their heads buried under the squashy surface.

These are some of the ways that a child can suffocate. The treatment for them all is basically the same.

WHAT TO LOOK FOR

The child will not have enough air to breathe and therefore not enough oxygen. If his body is deprived of oxygen completely for more than three minutes his brain cells will die, causing him brain damage and death.

● He may have difficulty in breathing – it may be noisy or 'gurgly'.

- He may froth at the mouth.

- He may look blue in the face, particularly around the mouth, nose and also the fingertips.

- He may be confused and not seem to recognise you.

- He may be unconscious.

- He may have stopped breathing altogether.

WHAT TO DO

- Get whatever it is that is stopping the child from breathing, away from him as soon as you possibly can. If it is sand, for instance, *uncover his mouth and nose first* to see if, just by doing that, he will start breathing again.

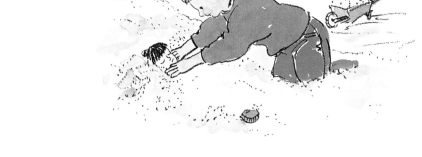

- Get the child into some fresh air, if he is not already outside, as soon as you can.

- If he is unconscious, open his airway and check his breathing. If breathing stops, start your ABC Resuscitation Routine as soon as you can.

> **A** for **AIRWAY**   (is it clear?)
>
> **B** for **BREATHING**   (is he breathing?)
>
> **C** for **CIRCULATION**   (is his heart beating?)

- Call for an ambulance by dialling 999 – if you can't do this, shout for attention and get someone else to do it. If you are on a beach, for instance, make sure whoever is calling for the ambulance gives precise directions as to where you are.

SUFFOCATION BY SMOKE

In a fire, the child is in great danger of suffocating, particularly if the room contains foam-filled furniture. You will want to try to get him out but unless you know exactly where he is in the room – and the chances are you won't – within minutes of entering you will die too. The fumes are lethal. Just before you go in after him *there are three things you MUST do*.

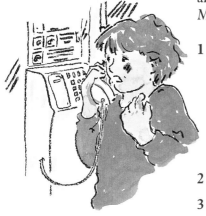

1 CALL THE FIRE BRIGADE by dialling 999. Tell them what you think has happened, as calmly as you can, and give them your address and telephone number (see Chapter 1 on Preparation and Practical Issues). Tell them that you think your child is trapped in a smoke-filled room and that you are going to try and get him out. *(They would prefer it if you didn't try this, but they will understand that you are probably going to have a go anyway.)*

2 Make sure that someone else knows you have gone into the room.

3 FEEL THE OUTSIDE DOOR-KNOB of the room with the back of your hand. (Or the door itself if it hasn't got a handle.) If the knob is hot to the touch DO NOT GO INTO THE ROOM. There is nothing you can do – it will be too late to save your child. If the heat of the room is enough to make that door-handle hot, he will not stand a chance of survival. If you open the door when the knob is hot and let oxygen into the room, the flames will just explode into a fireball, endangering you and anyone else who may be in the house or flat.

If, however, the door-knob is still cool, THIS IS WHAT YOU DO:

● Get help, then, if you can, tie something moist around your mouth and nose before you go into the room.

● However dark it is, DO NOT turn the light switch on or *strike a match* – it won't help you to see any more and it could cause an explosion.

● Don't walk, but GET DOWN ONTO YOUR STOMACH, so that your nose is almost in contact with the floor – the last 2 inches (5cm) nearest the floor *might* be free enough of smoke to let you reach the child. The lower you get, the safer you are and the greater your chances of getting him out.

● Try not to panic. Panicking will cause you to take an involuntary breath – that is, one which you didn't mean to take – and might make the difference between getting to the child or not.

● Unless you are sure where the child is lying – and the chances are you won't be – keep in contact with the wall and use it to guide you *from the moment you go through the door* (even if the room is very small). The carbon monoxide in the smoke will make you lose reason and mental control and you will become disorientated very quickly (after only a few seconds). *You can easily forget where the door is.* If you cannot cope with smoke or dark and confined spaces do *not* enter the room.

Children caught in fire tend to follow their animal instincts and hide from the flames. They will find somewhere to hide that looks 'safe', such as under the bed, in a cupboard, under the bedclothes, behind the sofa; and when the adult, in a panic, comes to search for them, they cannot be found.

So not only do you have the smoke to deal with, which can kill you very quickly if you don't take care, you have to think where in that room your child has crawled to hide. This is horrific but you must keep your wits about you. Think where he might be hiding *before* you go into the room. Children die in house fires every day, and more often than not they are found curled up in a place no one would have thought of looking.

WHAT TO DO

Once the child is away from the fire, this is what you do:

- CLOSE THE DOOR ON THE FIRE. If nobody has done so already, get someone to ring for the Fire Brigade and an ambulance, but otherwise leave the house or flat. If everyone is safely away from the fire, concentrate on saving the child's life.

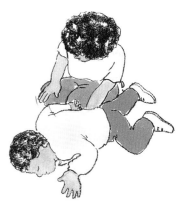

- Get him to some fresh air as quickly as you can (as long as he is not on fire). If your front door opens onto an indoor corridor, that will do, as long as he is well away from the fumes.

- If he is conscious put him in the Recovery Position in case he is sick. There is a possibility that the burnt lining of his throat may swell up and stop the child from breathing, so watch him very carefully.

- Reassure him as he will be terrified. Tell him that he is all right and everyone is safe, if that is the truth, otherwise just say that HE is safe; if he asks you about anyone else and you are not sure, say so.

- Don't leave him.

- If he is unconscious you must watch his breathing and if it stops, start your ABC Resuscitation Routine immediately.

> **A** for **AIRWAY**   (is it clear?)
>
> **B** for **BREATHING**   (is he breathing?)
>
> **C** for **CIRCULATION**   (is his heart beating?)

- Once you are sure his breathing is all right, check to see if he has any

251

burns (see Chapter 7 on Burns and Scalds) or any other injury. Don't forget to treat him for shock.

> ### REMEMBER – SHOCK LOOKS LIKE THIS
> - His face may be very pale and grey-looking
> - His skin may feel cold and clammy
> - His pulse may feel fast and weak
> - He may be frightened and fidgety
> - He may be very thirsty
> - He may yawn and 'gasp' for air
> - He may say everything feels fuzzy
> - He may become unconscious

- Get whatever it is that is stopping your child breathing away from his face as quickly as you possibly can – if it is sand or earth, scrape it away from his nose and mouth first. OR cut or tear away plastic bags from his face.
- Get the child into the fresh air as soon as you can.

THINK

- Have you managed to get some help? Try shouting out of the window or front door.
- Have you called the ambulance? Try to get someone to do this for you.
- Have you checked for DANGER?
- Shake and shout the child to see if he is conscious.

IF THE CHILD IS UNCONSCIOUS: be ready to start your ABC RESUSCITATION ROUTINE.

Now check 'A' for AIRWAY – is it clear?

OPEN THE AIRWAY. Tilt the child's head back and lift his chin forward. REMEMBER babies' necks are chubbier and more fragile. **Be gentle yet firm enough to tilt head back so airway is open.**

Now check 'B' for BREATHING

LOOK
LISTEN } for breathing
FEEL

IF THE CHILD IS NOT BREATHING: BREATHE FOR THE CHILD. Cover his mouth, or nose and mouth, with your mouth. Give him FIVE separate breaths. Watch his chest rise with each breath. REMEMBER you need *less* breath for babies.

Now check 'C' for CIRCULATION

Is his heart beating? Check for the pulse. Feel the neck (or arm in a baby) for a pulse. **If there is no pulse and you haven't got help GET IT NOW.**

IF YOU CANNOT FEEL A PULSE: DO CHEST COMPRESSION. Feel for the right place – one finger-breadth below the nipple line. Press on the chest, at a rate of **100 presses per minute.**

For children over one year old: Use the 'heel' of one hand only, with your arm straight. **Press fifteen times to every two breaths** (so your hand presses in about 2.5-3.5cm or 1-1½ inches each time).

For babies: Use two fingers only and **press five times to one breath** (so your fingers press in about 2cm which is about ¾ of an inch, each time).

KEEP DOING THIS UNTIL THE AMBULANCE ARRIVES.

29 SUICIDE

One-fifth of all emergency admissions to hospital are suicide attempts. The rate for boys over fifteen has doubled since 1982; the rate in other groups has stayed about the same but the numbers are huge, particularly among young people. One of the largest groups of people who contact the Samaritans are adolescent girls.

If your child has tried – or you feel *might* try – to harm herself in any way she (and you) will need special help.

If a young person takes an overdose of drugs and is sent to hospital, she may be thought of as a nuisance by the medical staff and felt to be 'wasting everyone's time' – although, as one counsellor says, 'It is quite obvious that people don't do it for fun.'

Suicide is the third largest cause of death in young people. What they need is for someone to try to find out why they want to do this. This means sitting down and listening to them. Some people find this difficult.

The Samaritans are an organisation committed to helping people to understand why they – or anyone, especially someone with their whole future before them – would even think about taking their own lives. They are beginning to set up workshops and training sessions for nurses and interested medical staff to look at the whole issue, particularly in young people.

There are also various Youth Projects being set up by Samaritan volunteers who go into schools and youth clubs to talk to children about life and death issues. They want to talk to young people about what it *feels* like to want to take your own life.

Something to remember is that nearly everyone who kills themselves *has spoken to someone about it within a month of their death*. In other words they meant what they said, but somehow there was no one there to listen.

If you are a parent whose child seems to have a 'suicide wish' your child (or you) might want to talk to the Samaritans. These hand-picked volunteers are specially trained to listen over the phone and they allow children to talk about their deepest fears.

They ask questions, or make the children question themselves, about why they think they would be better dead than alive. If the child wants to take it further but feels that it might be easier to talk face to face, she is asked if she would like to come into the office, where she is befriended by a volunteer until the immediate crisis is over. If, however, she would rather just chat to the same person again on the phone, she is invited to do this as many times as she wants to.

Any parent faced with the possibility that their child might take her own life is in a terrible situation. All you can do is to make her know how much you love her and to tell her you will do whatever it takes to make this awful situation better for her.

If you can, try and talk to her about it, confronting the issue of suicide and not shying away from it. Some of you may find this very difficult to do and if you can't, please don't feel guilty about it. Try and get a family friend, or your GP (if he is sensitive enough and feels he has the time it needs to tackle this) to talk to her, or give her the number of the Samaritans if she feels it would be easier to talk to a stranger.

If you feel you would like to try to talk to her there are one or two things that might help you make 'contact'. The first is to acknowledge that she is feeling dreadful – try not to fall into the trap of saying, 'I know how you must feel' or 'You really must try and pull your socks up' or 'Things can't be as bad as all that'. If in doubt say nothing – just listen.

You must let her see that, even if you have not done so in the past, you are now prepared to tackle the issue of her wanting to take her own life seriously.

Try to understand through gentle, patient, one-line questions, what she is feeling about her life and why she wants to end it all. When you feel able, ask her the question why she feels she would be better dead than alive – in other words, what's so special about being dead?

Be very aware that a child who is saying she is prepared to go to these desperate lengths will not be feeling very good about herself – her self-esteem and feelings of self-worth will be low. This may hurt you very much, especially if you feel that you have done all you possibly can for this child. But in order to help her now you have to try *not* to bring all this (the psychologists call it 'baggage') into the conversation. She may be doing it for all sorts of complex reasons – not the least of which is to get back at you in some way. Try not to respond angrily to anything she says – even though *she* may be angry with *you*.

The hardest thing for any parent to bear, however, is that if your child, for whatever reason, is determined to take her own life, she must be given the right to choose to do this. All you really can do is be there when she needs you.

Most adolescents who are thinking of taking their own lives will choose to take an overdose of drugs rather than choosing a method that is more certain to kill them because they are asking for help in some way. Those who are determined to die will throw themselves under a train or try something else from which there is no return.

You may miss the moment when she makes her move – depending on how serious she is. If she is going to take an overdose which is just a plea for help, it will be difficult for her to judge how to time it so that she gets medical help at the right time. Whatever she has taken, there is a possibility that she could lose consciousness and, of course, die.

- Once a child who has taken an overdose of drugs loses consciousness and cannot be roused, you must get medical help urgently. Don't wait to see if she loses consciousness. Call an ambulance by dialling 999 and tell them that you think your child has taken an overdose. Keep any containers of anything you think she might have taken.

- *Meanwhile watch the child carefully.* Young people who have taken an overdose of drugs and who have become unconscious, may go downhill rapidly.

- *Never assume that a child who is unconscious can't hear you.* She may lapse in and out of consciousness to find you doing things to her that might frighten her and make the situation worse. Talk to her gently and tell her everything that you are doing.

- Loosen any *tight clothing* either at her neck or waist as this will help her to breathe more easily.

- *If, at any time, you feel uneasy about her breathing* – maybe she is making a breathing noise as if something is stuck in her throat – put her in the Recovery Position, so that if she vomits there is less chance that she will inhale it. If you have a blanket or warm coat to hand, you may like to roll it under her.

- *Stay with the child all the time* and check her breathing and pulse at frequent intervals.

- NEVER try to give an unconscious child anything to eat or drink, even the smallest sip of water – she will just choke.

- If your child has cut her wrists (or any other part of her body), try to deal with her calmly, sympathetically but firmly. Stop the bleeding as soon as you can by direct pressure (see Chapter 6 on Bleeding). If she is in shock – she might be if she has lost a lot of blood – treat it quickly.

REMEMBER – SHOCK LOOKS LIKE THIS

- Her face may be very pale and grey-looking
- Her skin may feel cold and clammy
- Her pulse may feel fast and weak
- She may be frightened and fidgety
- She may be very thirsty
- She may yawn and 'gasp' for air
- She may say everything feels fuzzy
- She may become unconscious

● If she stops breathing, roll her out of the Recovery Position onto her back and start your ABC Resuscitation Routine immediately.

> **A** for **AIRWAY**   (is it clear?)
>
> **B** for **BREATHING**   (is she breathing?)
>
> **C** for **CIRCULATION**   (is her heart beating?)

● When the ambulance arrives *make sure you take any medicine containers, or pills you found near her, with you to the hospital*. It will help them to find an antidote to the 'poison' that she has taken.

Organisations that can help

You may need some support – but you may feel unable to share this situation with friends or family. There are a variety of organisations which have been set up to help parents find the courage to deal with difficult situations.

Parentline is run by parents for parents. It is a twenty-four hour service (after 5 p.m. there is an answerphone which will tell you the number of a volunteer you can speak to). There are twenty-five branches throughout the country. If there isn't one in your town, you can ring this central number for your nearest branch. The telephone number is:

Parentline 0268 757077

Parents Anonymous provide 'a sympathetic ear'. They stress they are not trained counsellors but will listen to problems and point parents in the direction of local organisations which will be able to give special help and support. Their telephone number is:

Parents Anonymous 071 263 8918

Parents and carers should be aware that children who try to harm themselves, or take their own lives, may have been physically or sexually abused. (See Chapter 26 on Sexual Abuse.)

If for any reason you are worried about a child being sexually abused, or even if *you* have been abused in this or any other way as a child, you might like to contact a new organisation set up by the NSPCC, called the NSPCC Child Protection Helpline. It is a twenty-four-hour confidential counselling service, run by qualified social workers for anyone who might want to get help or ask advice about child sexual abuse. The Freefone telephone number is:

NSPCC Child Protection Helpline 0800 800 500

The NSPCC also have a helpful leaflet for parents and carers called 'Protect Your Child'. You can send for it to this address:

NSPCC 67 Saffron Hill, London EC1N 8RS.

If you feel that a troubled child you know might like to talk to someone *in total confidence* on the telephone, he or she should ring Childline. This is a free twenty-four-hour service. The switchboard operator will transfer him or her to a trained counsellor. It is sometimes difficult to get through to Childline because so many children phone in, but he or she *will* get through eventually. The Freefone telephone number is:

Childline 0800 1111

OR the child might like to write in confidence to Childline. The address (no stamp needed) is:

Childline, Freepost 1111, London N1 0BR.

You may like to suggest to your child that she calls the Samaritans. They are *the* service devoted to those people for whom taking their own lives seems the only way out. It is a twenty-four hour telephone 'listening' service staffed by selected volunteers who have been specially trained to understand and help those driven to this final despair. There are 186 branches up and down the country. All the calls are in total confidence. Your child can ring, write or visit your local branch – the nearest one to you will be in your phone book.

For more information write to:

The Samaritans General Office
10 The Grove, Slough, SL1 1QP.

If you have a child who has tried to take her own life, or you have lost a child through suicide, you may find it helpful to contact the SOS (Shadow of Suicide) section of The Compassionate Friends. TCF (which is what they call themselves) is an international voluntary organisation, run by bereaved parents, which offers friendship and understanding, and provides one-to-one chats or contacts with other bereaved parents in your area. They also have a quarterly newsletter. Their address is:

The Compassionate Friends
6 Denmark Street, Bristol BS1 5DQ.
Tel. 0272 292778

The TCF recommend the following books: *Dear Stephen* by Ann Downey (a letter diary written to Stephen by his mother) (Arthur James Publishers); *Every Parents' Guide to Understanding Teenagers and Suicide: How to Recognise the Hidden Signs* by Marian Crooks (International Self Council Press, Canada); and *A Special Scar* by Alison Wertheimer (Routledge).

TWISTED TESTICLE, UNDESCENDED TESTICLE AND HERNIA

TWISTED TESTICLE

A boy's testicle can twist on its own and has rarely anything to do with the child playing with himself. This is one of the most painful experiences the child will ever have – even more painful than being *kicked* in the groin.

A TWISTED TESTICLE IS AN EMERGENCY.

If you don't act quickly and get the child to hospital he can lose the testicle. The twisting cuts off the blood supply and it has to be untwisted – by a doctor – as soon as possible. DO NOT try to do this yourself or let the child try to do it – it will only cause more injury.

WHAT TO LOOK FOR

- The child suddenly starts to roll around in pain, clutching his groin. He may also feel a severe pain at the bottom of his abdomen.

- If he lets you look at the testicle you will see that it is red-looking and swollen.

- He may feel violently sick or be sick.

- He will almost certainly be in shock.

WHAT TO DO

- You need to get him to hospital as quickly as possible. Call for an ambulance by dialling 999. Tell them what has happened.

- Treat him for shock (see Chapter 27 on Shock).

- You need to take the pressure off his lower abdomen and groin as much as you can. The way to do this is to gently lift his legs (you would do this to treat shock anyway) and gently put his head on a pillow.

● Reassure him. This child will be in a lot of pain and will be very frightened. The sound of your voice and your being there with him (after you have called the ambulance) will soothe him. Talk to him gently and tell him that help is on its way.

● DON'T give him anything to eat or drink. As soon as he gets to hospital he will probably need a small operation to untwist the testicle and fix it in place.

UNDESCENDED TESTICLE

If you notice that your son *looks* as if he only has one testicle (ball) in his scrotum (the sac that holds them) *then he has*.

It is important that once you discover this you take him to a doctor as soon as you can. He will then refer your child to the hospital where he will have to have a minor operation. This is done under general anaesthetic but he should be in and out in a day.

The earlier this is done the better and it should always have been seen to before the child goes to school to avoid his being teased. The other reason to have it done is to ensure the future generations of your family!

HERNIA

This is when there is a weak spot in the groin or around the tummy button. It can occur in boys and girls. You will see a lump sticking out which shouldn't be there – it is more obvious when the child is crying.

If you see any lump or bump that you think is unusual in your child, or if he has any peculiar pains 'down there', don't hesitate to take him to the doctor. He would much rather see a child unnecessarily, than not see a child who really does need medical attention.

- This child needs medical treatment urgently. Call for an ambulance by dialling 999. Tell them what has happened.
- Take pressure off his lower tummy and groin by *gently* lifting his legs and putting pillows or cushions underneath them. Then lift his head gently onto a pillow too.
- Reassure and comfort the child – he will be in a lot of pain.
- DO NOT give him anything to eat or drink.
- Treat the child for shock.

31 UNCONSCIOUSNESS

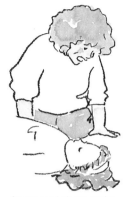

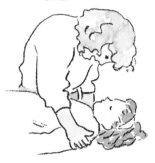

Shake and shout at the child.

A child who becomes unconscious will appear to be in a deep sleep and will be unaware of her surroundings. This is because the activity of her brain has been interrupted (probably temporarily) and she can no longer behave 'normally'. It may be difficult for you to understand what has happened but, however upset you may be at finding her in this situation, you must try and find out how deeply unconscious she is.

You have to do this in stages. You need to know your child's response to:

SOUND (your voice)

TOUCH (shaking her gently)

If there is some response, at either of these stages, the unconsciousness may be only light, but the danger is that she may sink into deeper unconsciousness very quickly.

If there is no response then she is deeply unconscious and the brain activity is dangerously depressed. She could stop breathing at any moment (although she may not) so you must be prepared to start your ABC Resuscitation Routine.

A for **AIRWAY**   (is it clear?)

B for **BREATHING**   (is she breathing?)

C for **CIRCULATION**   (is her heart beating?)

One of the most difficult things to deal with as a parent or carer of a child is understanding *why* the child has become unconscious. It is somehow easier if you know exactly what has happened.

However at this moment she IS unconscious (you can find out why later) and you will have to work quickly to give her the first aid she needs to keep her safe until she reaches hospital.

WHAT TO DO

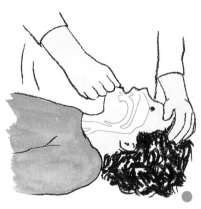

● Open her *airway* and check that it doesn't close again if she moves around. (Just because she is unconscious doesn't mean that she will lie still.) Being unconscious, especially deeply unconscious, means that she can't keep her own airway open.

● Make sure nothing is interfering with her *breathing* (such as a blocked-up nose or because her airway is closed).

● Look in her *mouth* to see if there is anything blocking her airway such as a piece of food, a bead, small toy or a sweet. (There would usually be clues to this in the place where you found her, like sweet wrappers or evidence of food – but there may not be.) If you think you see something do a quick 'finger-sweep'. DO NOT prod or poke: you may push whatever it is further down into the airway and block it.

● If you think she may have choked on something, turn her over your knee so that her head is well down and give five sharp slaps on the back, between the shoulder blades. See if anything comes flying out of her mouth after each slap. (See Chapter 8 on Choking.)

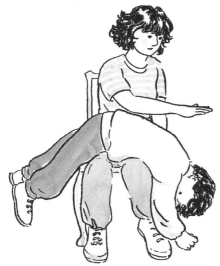

● Loosen any tight clothing at her neck or waist as this will help her to breathe more easily.

● *Watch her level of consciousness* (her breathing and her pulse). Occasionally an unconscious child will deteriorate quickly and may suddenly stop breathing, in which case you will have to breathe for her – so be prepared to start your ABC Resuscitation Routine.

If at any time you feel uneasy about her breathing WHETHER SHE HAS INJURIES OR NOT – maybe she is making a breathing noise, as if something is stuck in her throat – roll her into the Recovery Position, so that if she is sick there is less chance that she will inhale it and block her airway. If you have a blanket or warm coat to hand, you may like to roll it underneath her.

   If she stops breathing, quickly roll her out of the Recovery Position onto her back, check her airway and start your ABC Resuscitation Routine.

- Check to see if there is any obvious serious injury such as bleeding or fractures.

- Put direct pressure on any serious wound that is bleeding badly to prevent further blood loss (see Chapter 6 on Bleeding).

- Support any fractures as best you can, moving her as little as possible (see Chapter 18 on Fractures and Bone Injuries).

- Call an ambulance, by dialling 999, if you haven't managed to get someone to do this for you already, and stay with the child at all times until the ambulance arrives. Check her breathing and pulse at frequent intervals.

- NEVER try to give an unconscious child anything to eat or drink, even the smallest sip of water – she will choke.

- ALWAYS assume that your child can hear you *even if she can't respond*. Talk calmly and lovingly to her and tell her what you are doing so that she knows you are there. She may drift in and out of consciousness although you may not notice. When she does, it is important that she hears your voice and knows that you are there to take care of her.

Check the child's response to:

SOUND – shout 'Are you OK?'
TOUCH – shake her gently

IF THE CHILD DOESN'T RESPOND, SHE IS UNCONSCIOUS: be ready to start your ABC RESUSCITATION ROUTINE.

THINK

- Have you got help? Try shouting out of the window or front door.
- Have you called the ambulance? Try to get someone to do this for you.
- Have you checked for DANGER?

START YOUR ABC RESUSCITATION ROUTINE.

Now check   'A' for AIRWAY – is it clear?

IF SHE DOESN'T RESPOND: OPEN THE AIRWAY. Tilt the child's head back and lift her chin forward. REMEMBER babies' necks are chubbier and more fragile. **Be gentle yet firm enough to tilt head back so airway is open.**

Now check   'B' for BREATHING

LOOK
LISTEN } for breathing
FEEL

IF THE CHILD IS NOT BREATHING: BREATHE FOR THE CHILD. Cover her mouth, or nose and mouth, with your mouth. Give her FIVE separate breaths. Watch her chest rise with each breath. *Less* breath for babies.

Now check   'C' for CIRCULATION

Is her heart beating? Check for the pulse. Feel the neck or arm (in a baby) for pulse. **If there is no pulse and you haven't got help GET IT NOW.**

IF YOU CANNOT FEEL A PULSE: DO CHEST COMPRESSION. Feel for the right place – one finger-breadth below the nipple line. Press on the chest, at a rate of **100 presses per minute.**

For children over one year old: Use the 'heel' of one hand only, with your arm straight. **Press fifteen times to every two breaths** (so your hand presses in about 2.5-3.5cm or 1-1½ inches each time).

For babies: Use two fingers only and **press five times to one breath** (so your fingers press in about 2cm or about ¾ of an inch, each time).
KEEP DOING THIS UNTIL THE AMBULANCE ARRIVES.

If you feel the child may have choked on something:

- Have a look to see if anything obvious is blocking her airway. If you can see something, do a quick 'finger-sweep' to see if you can get it out. DO NOT push or probe. Turn her over and *give five sharp slaps on her back.* Check to see if anything comes flying out of her mouth.
- If she stays unconscious but is breathing, roll into the Recovery Position.

32 PREVENTING ACCIDENTS

Parents have to *think safe*. That doesn't mean to say it's the parents' fault if things go wrong and a child has an accident. You can't keep your eyes on the little dears twenty-four hours a day! What you can do, however, is to make the area inside and outside the home as safe as you can, be aware of the dangers, and know the people to whom you can turn if you need help.

Child safety is not *just* common sense. You really need to know what is safe and what isn't. Unfortunately one of the ways of finding out is by getting it wrong and having an accident! Another way is to share experiences with other parents, particularly those whose children are just slightly older than yours. (You can pass on your experience when it's someone else's turn to learn from you!) Try not to drive yourself crazy with anxiety – all you can do is be aware, and take sensible precautions.

THE FACTS

Accidents are the commonest cause of death in children. Three million children go to hospital each year having had an accident – out of these, about 120,000 are badly injured enough to have to stay in. Many more are treated by their GPs. About three children die in accidents every day.

Many accidents happen in the home, and research has shown that home accidents for all age groups happen mostly in the summer months – the highest rate is in July – and mostly on Sunday in the evening!

Most home accidents happen when the child is between one and four years old. It is the child's interest in the everyday articles that are around him that changes as he starts to grow. One day that trailing kettle flex and the cupboard under the sink with the cleaning fluids are fine, because 'he wouldn't go near them', the next, he wants to know more about them – and the everyday article becomes a hazard and he is in real danger.

Another major hazard, of course, is a busy road. Boys between the ages of five and eight years are most at risk of having a road accident, especially in the hours after school and before bed (3p.m.–9p.m.). Children under eight years should not be sent off to school or the shops by themselves if there are busy roads to cross – they are just too young to be aware of the dangers.

Children are just not totally reliable in traffic (on foot) until they are *twelve* and even then, not necessarily when they have just bought an ice-cream!

Children are naturally curious, have masses of energy and imagination, and want to explore all of their surroundings. It isn't to do with being naughty, it is just to do with wanting to know more. We as parents tend to think of our children as 'standing still' as far as their development is concerned. We are always amazed when they pull themselves up on their feet for the first time or put something in their mouths or begin to say things, as if we weren't somehow expecting it. Discuss what your child is capable of doing, at any particular age, with your Health Visitor. It is really important that you are one jump ahead of your child to work out what he *might* do – *before he does it!*

WHY ACCIDENTS HAPPEN

Accidents happen when parents, particularly women (as we tend to carry the brunt of the caring), are over-stressed and over-stretched – that must come as no surprise seeing that most of us do at least ten thousand jobs at the same time as looking after the kids. But this is only part of the story.

Parents have to ask themselves what changes they could make or what changes they wish they had made (if their child has had an accident) to be sure their home is safe. It could be something as simple as putting child-locks on the 'poisons' cupboard or catches on the upstairs windows or even making patio doors/French windows shatter-proof. And children need to understand at as early an age as possible the importance of keeping safe.

Little children are not aware of danger – they just don't have the experience to be able to tell which things can harm them and which are OK. They cannot tell the difference, for instance, between unpleasant-tasting, dangerous substances and safe foods until they are about three. They cannot judge the place or speed of a car on the road as it comes zooming towards them.

WHAT YOU CAN DO TO TEACH YOUR CHILD ABOUT SAFETY

You still have to be on your guard, but once your child is four, at least you can begin to *explain* to him why he mustn't do the things he is doing.

There are lots of 'do's and don'ts' to tell children about preventing accidents, but they also need to be told *why* they should or shouldn't do these things, so that they can understand the reasons behind the advice. Everyone needs to understand why they are being told something, particularly when it seems to be important, and children are no different.

267

Parents also need to understand why their children *want* to do the things they do – we need to try to see things more through their eyes. Recently children were asked what safety meant to them. They had a general idea about things like 'accidents' and 'danger', especially if they themselves had had some sort of horrid experience. To some children 'safety' also meant things like making a mistake, breaking something, talking to strangers ('stranger danger') and possible racial attacks, as well as safety in the home.

There are lots of excellent books already written about the 'do's and don'ts' and any of these, read together and discussed, can really help to get safety messages across. But it is important how you get the information across to your child. If you ask many young children what they should or shouldn't do in any given situation, they will probably repeat to you (parrot fashion) what they have been told, but put them in a real situation and they may act very differently – which shows they have listened but not really *understood*. For instance, an interesting piece of research, done recently on childhood accidents, has shown that kerb drill was seen by children to be enough in itself to keep them safe – in other words they thought that by looking 'right and left and right again' they wouldn't have an accident. The drill wasn't done to *see* the car coming, just to stop the car hitting them – rather like a magic spell!

How can parents possibly know, therefore, what on earth is in a child's mind and what his brain will do with the information that goes in. It's rather like a cement mixer – you put in three ingredients and out comes something quite different. At least with a cement mixer you know what to expect the other side – with a child you don't!

Perhaps we have to 'package' the information so that the child can see the situation from various points of view. Road safety, for instance, can be tackled from outside (crossing the road), and inside (from a car or bus), so that he can see different sides of the problem. The more he is told the information in as many different forms as possible, the more he is going to understand.

By far the best way to teach children anything is by discussion. This takes time – a luxury not many of us have. The information has to have the 'why' (you do things) built into it, as well as the 'what' (you want him to do). The other trick – rather an old one – is to praise and reward any information that actually sticks in his mind (remember it is more *how he acts*, than what he says that is important), rather than telling him off if he gets it wrong. The final thing that might help to keep his interest and (hopefully) enthusiasm going, is for him to take part in safety competitions – the school might be interested in this.

The one thing *parents* have to do (boring though it may be) is to set a good example – in other words do the things you tell the children to do. It is easy to forget how much our children are always looking at us to see what we are doing and how we are behaving in any given situation. They just soak it all up like sponges.

GETTING HELP

In 1989 the Children Act came into force. It is – as far as the Child Accident Prevention Trust is concerned – '*the* most important piece of legislation on behalf of children this century'. Keeping children safe is an important part of the Act and parents should be offered support, information and guidance on accident prevention.

What parents need, to make and keep their child safe, is lots of understanding and support. Every parent needs help at some time and getting child safety right is difficult to do by yourself. Ask your Health Visitor – she is the one person who will come to your home and discuss this with you. Maybe you have never met yours (if, for instance, you moved into an area when your children were no longer very little) but once you have registered with your GP, she will want to come and meet you anyway.

But there are other ways, apart from chatting with your Health Visitor. Don't knock mother and toddler groups – you may not be able to get to one, because you are working, or the times don't suit you, but try to find one to go to. There's nothing like it – just to have a moan, apart from anything else, and to talk to other mothers who may also be finding it tough. (Mother and toddler groups are also an excellent starting point to get together to start pressurising the local council – or whoever is responsible – about the safety standards, or lack of them, in your local playground.) If you are a single parent, or you are short of money, looking after a child is going to be that much tougher, particularly if you don't have a mum around the corner to give *you* a cuddle when things get too much!

The need to let children take risks

The most natural thing in the world for a parent to want to do is to protect a child from danger. But it is just as important to let children take risks so that they learn safely, when they are ready. If you wrap them up in cotton wool and don't go with their natural need to explore, they could become too over-protected and lack the confidence to be on their own – and these children are more likely to have a *major* accident than a minor one.

MAKING YOUR HOME SAFE

There are some things to do to make your child safe that the 'experts' feel are absolute musts. These include:

Smoke alarms

These are very reassuring things to have in your home – they let you know as soon as there is any smoke around it so that you can act

269

Make sure all safety products have the kite mark (always check safety equipment).

RESISTANT

Check all furniture, furnishings and clothes for a *fire resistant* label.

quickly and get the family out of the house. Placing one upstairs and one downstairs – or just the one if you are all on one level – will warn you if there is a fire in your home. These can be bought very cheaply. The prices differ depending on where you buy them, but the cheaper ones are fine – as long as you look for the 'kite' mark of the BSI (British Standards Institute) which shows it has been tested for safety and reliability. (Don't forget to read the instructions carefully: if you don't put the alarms in the right place, they won't do the job they are supposed to do – they have to be fitted *high up* because smoke rises.)

Fire blankets

This is very important to have in the kitchen. It acts by smothering the flames and closing off the air (and therefore the oxygen). Without oxygen, the fire just goes out. It is extremely comforting to know that one of these is handy just in case something you are cooking starts to get too hot and catches fire.

Stair gates

Stairs without protection are dangerous to small children, even those past the toddling stage because they cannot know how steep they are, or judge the distance to the top of the stairs from where they may be playing on the landing.

Stair gates must have a snug fit with the walls on either side of the stairs and must be 'kite' marked for safety. They must be easily removable in case of fire but firm enough to hold a sturdy ten-month-old as he tries to stand, using the safety gate to test his muscle! (Don't be afraid to let your child learn the necessary skill of going up and down stairs – after a few 'safe' tumbles, you and he will feel more confident.)

Fire guards, plug covers and cupboard locks

These will help you to feel more confident and less anxious if you and your child move around your home in different directions at the same time! You cannot keep your eye on your child twenty-four hours a day and the moment that your back is turned is *the* moment he will get it in his head to put that nice shiny screw-driver he found in the cupboard into one of those three small holes he can see in the wall.

General precautions

Remember, most accidents are preventable, but no parent or carer can watch a child every minute of every day. *You have to get into the 'safety habit'*. Here are a few 'do's' you might want to think about:

- *Always* turn pan handles in so a child cannot reach up and pull the boiling liquid down over himself.

- *Always* shorten kettle flexes – for the same reason. (So many children get scalded in this way by pulling the kettle down on top of themselves.)

270

● *Always* lock away medicines and anything that might be poisonous to a child (in one year recently, *nearly 9000 three-to-four-year-olds were poisoned at home*).

● *Always* put away equipment 'dangerous' to a child and mend loose plugs and leads.

But please remember, it is not just *your* home that you need to be aware of – it's other people's as well. This is the most difficult thing of all, particularly with friends or your parents. ALL you can do is be aware that they *don't* have window catches on the upstairs windows for instance, or that they have a pond at the bottom of the garden, or *don't* lock up their 'poisons' in the cupboard under the sink. Try to find a way to broach the subject that isn't going to hurt feelings but should keep your child safe.

However, there is one thing that all those associated with child safety are in agreement about – *the absolute danger of baby walkers*. DO NOT BUY ONE – they are lethal. Using one of these things is like putting a baby on roller skates. Babies are not supposed to be able to get very far very quickly, that's why their legs are made the way they are! Once you put wheels on them they just steer themselves into danger. If you have a baby walker and you can afford to do this, *get rid of it.*

Many parents worry about the expense of safety equipment. There may be a loan/hire scheme in your area to help you get the equipment you feel you need to keep your child safe – especially if you are on a low income. Ask your Health Visitor if she knows where the nearest loan scheme is in your area. If there isn't one near you perhaps you could persuade her to start one. You may have to rally a group of parents to support her – but once in operation, parents find these schemes invaluable.

SAFETY FOR CHILDREN IN PUBLIC PLACES

Government bodies have an important role in supporting and working with parents to keep children as safe as possible in the environment in which they live.

There is a lot of pressure being put on the Government at the moment by organisations like the Royal Society for the Prevention of Accidents (ROSPA) and the Child Accident Prevention Trust to change the laws about safety standards and reduce the appalling number of accidents happening to children.

There are three major changes that have so far saved thousands of children's lives. Children have to 'belt up' in the back of cars. As Esther Rantzen once said on *That's Life*, 'You wouldn't let fragile china loose on the back seat of your car, so why let your children?' Shortly afterwards the Government brought in the legislation to make the wearing of seat belts in the back seats compulsory. Children are also now advised to wear bicycle helmets when cycling on the road, and the use of child-resistant medicine containers has (hopefully) changed child poisoning statistics for ever. They have dropped dramatically.

Playground safety (or lack of it) is causing great concern to a lot of parents. It is amazing how different some playgrounds are from one area to another. *All playgrounds should be safe for children to play in*, but it is often in well-to-do areas that children seem to have the safest, nicest, most brightly painted, most sensibly designed places to play. Perhaps low-income parents just don't have the time or energy to make a fuss about appalling play conditions and local councils know this and sometimes take advantage of it.

Each year about 150,000 children are injured in playground accidents. Four out of every five of these happen even though the children *are being supervised.*

If you live in an older local authority (council) flat or housing estate, the architects and planners may not have thought through the best way to keep your children safe. Safety wasn't thought to be as important then as it is now. Councils are now rethinking how to make local authority property as safe as possible for children, in spite of serious underfunding.

If you are worried that the area your child plays in is not as safe as you would like, you may want to start by making a general enquiry at your local town hall. Ask for the Under Eights' Advisor who is now dealing with your local play facilities about whatever it is that is worrying you. (Since the introduction of the Children Act in 1989, there will be someone who has special responsibility for this – it could be within the leisure, education or community services departments.) Ask to speak to the director of that department and don't be fobbed off with anyone less than that. You will find that everyone now, from the town hall information departments upwards, is keen to listen to parents' problems or anxieties about issues to do with children's play.

You may want to contact your ward councillor and get her (or him) onto your side. Tell her what the problem is and what you feel you should both be working towards.

You may want to lobby the Chair of your local leisure committee, or whichever committee it is that has the responsibility for children's play facilities.

You may want to approach your local school to see if you are able to use their playground and playground equipment during the school holidays, especially if you don't have many areas around you where your child can play.

Any or all of these things might be easier to do as part of a group. If there is more than one of you, you can spur one another on if the going gets tough, although you may find that all the people I've suggested are delighted to hear from you and really welcome your proposals.

Some local authorities plead poverty and say the reason that play areas are so bad in their borough is that there is no money – even though they agree that improvements should be made. Others in the same financial position think that improving children's play facilities is one of the *most important* public services that should be provided and they set about introducing long-term changes that guarantee that the children playing in their area are SAFE.

And it is not just a matter of providing any old playground. It is important that whatever new facilities are provided *match what is needed for that particular area*. In other words, there needs to be a detailed investigation into the age and sex of most of the children who live in that area and the *type* of play that the children want.

There are now new standards being set in Europe about child playground safety and, over the next few years, governments and local authorities will be bound by law to apply these to ALL areas in which children play.

The National Playing Fields Association is an important charity set up to campaign for and improve play facilities. They are a small caring organisation and, along with others, are committed to helping parents and carers fight for the right for a child to play safely.

These booklets might help: 'Playground Planning for Local Communities' and 'School Playgrounds'. Both are written for parents and both are published by:

The National Playing Fields Association
25 Ovington Square, London SW3 1LQ.
Tel. 071 584 6445

Another helpful booklet is 'Playground Safety Guidelines', written mainly for those who help to run children's playgrounds. It is published by:

The National Play and Recreation Unit
Welsh Office Education Department, Cathays Park, Cardiff CF1 3NQ.
Tel. 0222 823370

'Accident Prevention in Day Care and Play Settings', published by the Child Accident Prevention Trust, is a two-volume pack which includes a 'training resource' and 'practical guide' which together provide information to all those concerned with the issue of child day care and play safety. It costs £14.95 for the two, or £6.50 for just the practical guide, and is available from:

The Child Accident Prevention Trust
4th Floor, Clerk's Court, 18-20 Farringdon Lane, London EC1R 3AU.
Tel. 071 608 3828

You may feel that what is needed is to start a safety campaign. You may find this easier to do with other parents or your local mother and toddler group – your Health Visitor will advise you where it is. She will also tell you about other groups and organisations in your area, who might be able to help.

The following organisations are concerned with safe and adequate play facilities for children and will give you the advice and support you need to get your message across or your campaign started:

The National Children's Play and Recreation Unit
359-361 Euston Road, London NW1 3AL.
Tel. 071 383 5455

Play Wales
10/11 Raleigh Walk, Atlantic Wharf, Cardiff CF1 5LN.
Tel. 0222 498909

Play Board Northern Ireland
253 Lisburn Road, Belfast BT9 7EN.
Tel. 0232 382633

The National Centre for Play
Moray House College of Education, Cramond Campus, Cramond Road North, Edinburgh EH4 6JD.

You may also want to try:

The National Playing Fields Association
25 Ovington Square, London SW3 1LQ.
Tel. 071 584 6445

Alternatively, you could try your local Road or Home Safety Officer at your local council office or The Association for Consumer Research (see page 280 for their address). There are some other names and addresses of organisations at the end of the chapter that you might find useful.

OTHER ASPECTS OF KEEPING YOUR CHILD SAFE

There is one other aspect of preventing accidents to children that we haven't covered, and that is when things get so bad for you that you do something that in 'normal' circumstances you would not dream of doing.

Perhaps your child has been crying for the last hour and you are just too tired or depressed to do anything about seeing to *his* needs, when you need someone to see to *yours*. And then you snap. It is those moments when you need as much help and support as you can get, and no matter how awful you feel you *must* ask for help. Do not take your anger, frustration and pain out on your child – you will never forgive yourself if you do. Just walk away – even if it means leaving the child alone for a few minutes. In these circumstances, he is less at risk alone than he is from you harming him. Go and walk round the block, go into another room and scream, phone someone – anyone – as long as you trust them. Or phone the NSPCC Helpline just to talk through your pain (in complete confidence). There are other organisations who also have good 'ears' for situations like this – for instance Cry-Sis, a support group for mothers with crying babies (details below).

Please be aware of others who come into your home to look after your child. It will horrify you to know that I recently employed a mother's help who the children kept telling me they didn't like – but I was too busy to listen. Weeks after she left, they told me that on regular occasions she used to bend their fingers back, pinch their ears and was generally nasty to them. I just didn't have the time to really *hear* what they were saying.

Sometimes people who seek work with children may have problems left over from their own childhood. Child-minders should be registered; never allow children under sixteen years to babysit, unless they are your own; and if you employ anyone to look after your kids, either on a full-time or part-time basis, always ask for references and *follow them up with a telephone call*, to double check until you are satisfied.

Always tell the babysitter where you are going and leave a number where you can be reached. I always make a point of ringing halfway through the evening just to make sure everything is OK.

Kidscape is a nationwide charity which works for child safety, particularly the prevention of bullying, abduction (being taken away against their will) and physical and sexual abuse. Kidscape provides information to all carers as well as parents, including teachers, social workers, youth leaders and police.

They have written their own code for parents which I think is extremely helpful:

Kidscape Code for Parents

Children need to know how:

- *To be safe*. Teach children that everyone has rights, such as the right to breathe, which should not be taken away. Tell children that no one should take away their right to be safe.

- *To protect their own bodies*. Children need to know that their body belongs to them, particularly the private parts covered by their swim suits.

- *To say no*. Tell children it's all right to say no to anyone if that person tries to harm them. Most children are taught to listen to and obey adults and older people without question.

- *To get help against bullies*. Bullies usually pick on younger children. Tell children to enlist the help of friends or say no without fighting – and to tell an adult. Bullies are cowards and a firm, loud NO from a group of children with the threat of adult intervention often puts them off.

In cases of real physical danger, children often have no choice but to surrender to the bully's demand. Sometimes children will fight and get hurt to protect a possession because of the fear of what will happen when they arrive home without it. 'My mum will kill me for letting the bullies take my bike. It cost a lot of money.' Tell children that keeping themselves safe is the most important consideration.

- *To tell.* Assure your children that no matter what happens you will not be angry with them and that you want them to tell you of any incident. Children can also be very protective of parents and might not tell about a frightening occurrence because they are worried about your feelings.

- *To be believed.* When children are told to go to an adult for help, they need to know they will be believed and supported. Although sometimes an immediate reaction is to say 'I told you so', this will not help the child to resolve the problem. It could also prevent the child from seeking help another time.

  This is especially true in the case of sexual assault, as children very rarely lie about it. If the child is not believed when he or she tells, the abuse may continue for years and result in suffering and guilt for the child.

- *Not to keep secrets.* Teach children that some secrets should NEVER be kept, no matter if they promised not to tell. Child molesters known to the child often say that a kiss or touch is 'our secret'. This confuses the child who has been taught always to keep secrets.

- *To refuse touches.* Explain to children that they can say 'yes' or 'no' to touches or kisses from anyone, but that no one should ask them to keep touching a secret. Children sometimes do not want to be hugged or kissed, but that should be a matter of choice not fear. They should not be forced to hug or kiss anyone.

- *Not to talk to strangers.* It is NEVER a good idea to talk to a stranger. Since most well-meaning adults or teenagers do not approach children who are by themselves (unless the child is obviously lost or in distress), teach children to ignore any such approach. Children do not have to be rude – they can pretend not to hear and quickly walk or run away. Tell children you will never be angry with them for refusing to talk to strangers and that you want to know if a stranger ever talks to them.

  Be careful how you put all this across to your child. You never know when your child might have to turn to a stranger in an emergency and you don't want her to feel that all strangers are going to harm her.

- *To break rules.* Tell your children that they have your permission to break all rules to protect themselves and tell them you will always support them if they must break a rule to stay safe. For example, it is all right to run away, to yell and create a fuss, even to lie or kick to get away from danger.

Michele Elliott, Director of Kidscape, also has guidelines for parents with older children who wish to stay out late at night:

Staying out late

This is the perennial arguing point for many parents and children. What time is late? What time is fair? What time is bedtime? We think it's important that all of this is negotiated between you, but that you teach your child rules which will keep her safer when she's out at night. Tell your child:

- To tell you where she is going and who she is going with.

- All you are concerned about is her safety and if anything bad happens, even if she feels guilty or bad about it, she must still ring you, or someone you both know and trust who has a phone, and tell you where she is so you can come and get her.

- If there's a real need, she can get a taxi home and you will pay at the other end. And make sure she knows how to make a reversed charge phone call.

- You will all agree on a time she must be home and make sure she sticks to it.

- Whatever her friends say, she mustn't do anything she doesn't feel comfortable with. She doesn't have to give reasons – it is her right to refuse to take part in whatever they're doing.

- Whatever anyone says, her body is her own and she doesn't have to do anything she doesn't want to. (Daughters must know that even if they've kissed and cuddled with a boy it is their right to say that they don't want to go any further. A boy has no right to force a girl to do anything. She shouldn't believe him if he says she 'led him on'.)

- To stay together as a group – don't drift away from the pack.

- To use her instincts to tell her if the group is doing something she doesn't approve of – maybe taking a stolen car, maybe sniffing glue. If so, leave with anyone else who doesn't want to get involved.

- To keep away from unlit streets, yards and alleyways. If anything seems at all threatening, run for help to the nearest person or house with lights on. If anyone tries to steal anything from her, it's better to give it up if her safety is in danger.

- Don't hitchhike. And don't accept lifts from strangers.

- Keep away from places she knows may mean trouble, such as amusement arcades and rowdy cafés. Don't go into pubs.

RECOMMENDED READING

Reading books, or even really well-produced leaflets, together can help to get safety messages across.

Michele Elliott, Director of Kidscape, has written *Feeling Happy, Feeling Safe* (Hodder & Stoughton), which deals with all aspects of safety covered by these Codes, and *The Willow Street Kids* (Pan/Piccolo), which deals with bullying, 'stranger danger' and child abuse.

Kidscape also publish a twenty-page guide to 'Bullying' and a sixteen-page guide to 'Keeping Children Safe'. If you want either of these excellent *free* publications, send a stamped addressed envelope to:

Kidscape
152 Buckingham Palace Road, London SW1W 9TR.
Tel. 071 730 3300
(They get between *500 to 1000 letters and requests for information every week*, so it is really important to send an SAE!)

ROSPA (The Royal Society for the Prevention of Accidents) recommends *Playing Safe: The Parents' Guide to Children's Safety In and Out of the Home* by S. Sayer (Thorsons).

These are the publications recommended by the Child Accident Prevention Trust (address on facing page):

- *Play It Safe* is a BBC publication following on from the excellent television series of the same name. *Play It Safe* is also available on video.

- *You Can Say No*, by David Pithers and Sarah Green – about dealing with strangers trying to entice children into dangerous situations.

There are also some very good leaflets including 'Keep Your Baby Safe', 'Keep Them Safe', 'First Ride Safe Ride'. These are available from the Child Accident Prevention Trust and the Health Education Authority (address on facing page).

If your Health Visitor would like more information, the Child Accident Prevention Trust have written an excellent booklet as part of their 'Approaches to Child Accident Prevention Project'.

USEFUL CONTACTS

If you feel your building or your local play area is dangerous in any way to your kids, or if you want general safety information, here are some organisations who may be able to help:

The Child Accident Prevention Trust
4th Floor, Clerk's Court, 18-20 Farringdon Lane, London EC1R 3AU.
Tel. 071 608 3828

The Health Education Authority
Hamilton House, Mabledon Place, London WC18 9TX.
Tel. 071 383 3833

Here are some organisations that you may want to contact for more information or for help in a crisis:

Cry-Sis

Cry-Sis is an organisation set up for parents who are at their wits' end with their baby, either because he won't stop crying (or so it seems) or because he won't sleep. It is run by parents who have been through similar problems and who have then had special training to help them deal with desperate parents.

There is a twenty-four-hour telephone service and the number is:
Cry-Sis 071 404 5011

The switchboard operator will ask you *the name of the television area you live in*. She will then give you one or two numbers to contact, of people manning the phones in your area – whatever time of the day or night.

If you then join Cry-Sis (for a small membership fee) you get all sorts of literature, giving you checklists, for instance, of the sorts of things which might make your baby cry.

Parentline

Parentline is run by parents for parents. There are twenty-five branches throughout the country. If there isn't one in your town, you can ring this central number for your nearest branch. It is a twenty-four-hour service and the number is:
Parentline 0268 757077
(After 5 p.m. there is an answerphone which will tell you the number of a volunteer you can speak to.)

Parents Anonymous

Parents Anonymous provides 'a sympathetic ear'. They stress they are not trained counsellors but will listen to problems and point parents in the direction of local organisations which will be able to give specific help and support.

The telephone number is:
Parents Anonymous 071 263 8918

279

NSPCC

If you feel that *you* are out of control of any angry feelings that you have towards your child or children (by being violent or ill-treating them in some way) you may want to talk about it to someone, and you may need help. Or if you think that your child might be being generally ill-treated *within your family*, and you don't feel in control of the situation, or you are finding it difficult to face up to what is happening, it might help to talk to someone who will listen and will understand what you are going through.

In either of these situations, you might like to contact a new organisation set up by the NSPCC, called the NSPCC Child Protection Helpline. It is a twenty-four-hour confidential counselling service, run by qualified social workers for anyone who might want to get help or ask advice about child abuse.

The Freefone telephone number is:

NSPCC Child Protection Helpline 0800 800 500

The NSPCC also have a helpful leaflet for parents and carers called 'Protect Your Child'. You can send for it at this address:

NSPCC
67 Saffron Hill, London EC1N 8RS.

Association for Consumer Research
2 Marylebone Road, London NW1 4DX.
Tel. 071 486 5544
(Publish *Which?* magazine and *Which Way to Health?*)

British Standards Institution
Linford Wood, Milton Keynes MK14 6LE.
Tel. 0908 221166

Department of Trade and Industry
Consumer Safety Unit, 10-18 Victoria Street, London SW1H 0NN.
Tel. 071 215 3215

National Consumer Council
20 Grosvenor Gardens, London SW1W 0DH.
Tel. 071 730 3469

Royal Society for the Prevention of Accidents (ROSPA)
Cannon House, Priory Queensway, Birmingham B4 6BS.
Tel. 021 200 2461

St John Ambulance
1 Grosvenor Crescent, London SW1X 7EF.
Tel. 071 235 5231
(Your local branch will be in the telephone book)

Please don't forget that your GP and Health Visitor are always there to give you advice on any problems that are worrying you about your child.

FIRST AID KIT

In case of an emergency, it is important and comforting to know you have some sterile or clean equipment to keep the child as safe as you can, whilst you wait for medical help.

First aid kits have changed a great deal – they used to be big, bulky and complicated with lots of different bandages and dressings. Now they are simple and a lot more efficient. Triangular bandages are out! Scarves, shirts, jumpers do the same job, as do other limbs which can be used to keep injured limbs still. (See Chapter 18 on Fractures and Bone Injuries.)

The first thing to do in any accident is to make sure the child's airway is open and that she is breathing. Do this BEFORE you look after a wound of any sort. (See Chapter 3 on ABC Resuscitation Routine.)

Now see to the injuries – please look under the chapter for each particular injury to see what you have to do. Generally, however:

- Minor bleeding has to be *cleaned and covered*.

- Major bleeding has to be *stopped by direct pressure* as quickly as you can with fingers or clean covering first, then dressings whenever someone can pass them to you or you can get them yourself.

- Burns must be *cooled and then covered* only with something clean (or ideally sterile).

Children get very frightened when they hurt their bodies in any way – it's not just making a fuss. They need to be comforted and cuddled with even quite minor injuries. There seems something magical about a plaster that seems to calm the most distraught child.

There is a story we read in our house, called *On the Way Home* by Jill Murphy, about a little girl called Claire who hurts her knee. The book is about the fantasmagorical tales Claire tells her friends about *how* she hurt her knee. At the end of the story, however, she arrives home and for the first time bursts into tears. Her mum comforts her and says she'll put a plaster on it. Claire asks for a 'very BIG plaster' and her mum replies, 'The biggest in the whole box'! Well, I can't tell you the satisfaction this last line brings to our kids. It's like the best thing that could possibly happen if you have hurt yourself . . .

So what are the most important and useful items to have in any first aid kit in the home? (It is also useful to carry one in the car and a little one in a rucksack or carrier bag if you go out for the day.)

WHAT YOU NEED

- *Cotton wool* (one 15gm packet). Any graze or wound that is not bleeding too much could do with a gentle wash (not burns – they are already sterile). Cool water is the best thing to get out little bits of gravel and dirt using the cotton wool. Only use the cotton wool *after you have washed your hands* and never use the same piece of cotton wool twice.

- *Antiseptic* to clean the wound. Antiseptic wipes are great but are expensive and wasteful. You just wipe around the wound once and throw it away. If the wound is still dirty, use another one.

- *Plasters* (a box of assorted fabric dressings or fabric strip). Personally I don't like waterproof plasters. They tend to make the wound 'sweat' and so it doesn't heal as quickly as it could. A lot of people disagree. I also prefer a strip of plaster rather than the box of assorted ones – even though they are not sterile – because I can never find the right size that I need. I put the biggest one on and then I'm left with all the small ones at the end of the packet.

- *Dressings* (two medium-sized ones). These now come as an all-in-one dressing and bandage. All you have to remember is to unravel it carefully so that the whole lot doesn't drop on the floor! (These are also excellent in their rolled-up state to support either side of an object that is stuck in a wound so that it doesn't do any further damage until the child gets to hospital. The whole wound is then bandaged firmly *on either side of* the object. See Chapter 6 on Bleeding.)

- *Bandages* (one each of 5cm and 7.5cm). You may want a bandage but no dressing (see above). Crêpe bandages have been replaced by retention bandages because they are cheaper. They come in fine, light stretchy gauze-type material and pack up very small.

- *Non-stick sterile dressings* (one each of 5cm square and 10cm square). These are ideal for burns. Please remember, *burns have to be cooled first* for at least TEN MINUTES before putting on any dressing. Don't move a child injured in this way until you have covered the burnt area – burns get infected very quickly. It is more difficult to do any grafting or surgery on an infected burn. (See Chapter 7 on Burns and Scalds.)

- *Large sticky-plaster dressings* (two 8.3cm by 6cm). This is for any wound other than a burn. NEVER put a sticky dressing on a burn. When you pull the dressing off, you could injure the child more by pulling off peeling skin.

- *Eye-pad*. This is useful for covering the eyes if they are injured, or for a child to bite on when she has a bleeding tooth socket that refuses to stop bleeding.

- *A pair of scissors*, for cutting plaster strips or bandage.

● *Six safety pins* for pinning up and supporting broken limbs in jumpers, scarves, etc. (see Chapter 18 on Fractures and Bone Injuries) or for fastening bandages in place.

St John Ambulance has a large variety of 'standard' first aid kits. These kits contain all the *essential* things you would need if your child had an accident. It will save you having to think of all the bits and pieces that you need. There are, however, some things you can add to (or keep near) your basic first aid kit:

● *Antiseptic cream.* Serious first aiders, like St John, would say you don't need it. But children do like to have something soothing to put on a sore place (as well as a plaster) and it does help to make them feel better.

● *Eye-wash bottle or feeding cup.* Either of these are very useful to splash water into a child's eye or onto a burn.

● *'Bump pack'.* This is a small pouch into which you can put a block of ice. It is made out of material of some kind such as flannel, and is used when a child bumps himself. Ours is shaped like a teddy's head and is called the 'teddy bump pack'. Ice is the best thing to stop children bruising and swelling up when they bump themselves, as long as it's held on long enough. It is more likely to stay on longer in one of these packs because it is more 'child friendly' than ice-cubes or a packet of peas!

● *Arnica cream.* This is the next best thing to ice – the two together are great. Arnica is a homoeopathic cream made especially to relieve the pain of bruising and stop it from turning black. You rub it onto the bump immediately after it has been cooled with the ice for at least five minutes.

BIBLIOGRAPHY AND RECOMMENDED READING

Bibliography

Elliott, Michele, *Keeping Safe: A Practical Guide to Talking with Children*, New English Library, 1988.

Pease, K. & Preston, B., 'Road Safety Education for Young Children', *British Journal of Educational Psychology*, 1967.

Sibert, Professor Jo, 'Accidents to Children: the Doctor's Role', *Education or Environmental Change*.

Recommended Reading List

Buchanan, Neil, *Childhood Asthma*, London, Judy Piatkus, 1987.

Crisp, Arthur, *Anorexia Nervosa: Let Me Be*, London, Baillière Tindall, 1990.

Crooks, Marian, *Every Parent's Guide to Understanding Teenagers and Suicide: How to Recognise the Hidden Signs*, Canada, International Self Council Press, 1988.

Downey, Ann, *Dear Stephen*, London, Arthur James Publishers, 1987.

Elliott, Joanne, *If Your Child is Diabetic*, London, Sheldon Press, 1987.

Elliott, Michele, *Feeling Happy, Feeling Safe*, London, Hodder & Stoughton, 1991.

Elliott, Michele, *The Willow Street Kids*, London, Piccolo, 1990.

Estridge, Bonnie, and Davies, Jo, *So Your Child has Diabetes?*, London, Vermilion, 1992.

Gold, Milton, and Zimmerman, Barry, *Allergies and Children*, Cambridge, CUP, 1989.

Hillson, Rowan, *Diabetes: A Young Person's Guide*, London, Optima, 1988.

Levene, Sara, *Play It Safe: The Complete Guide to Child Accident Prevention*, London, BBC Books, 1992.

Parsons, Alexandra and Iain, *Making it from 12-20: How to Survive Your Teens*, London, Judy Piatkus, 1991.

Patterson, Claire, and Quilter, Lindsay, *It's OK to be You: Feeling Good about Growing Up*, London, Piccolo, 1991.

Pithers, David, and Greene, Sarah, *We Can Say No*, London, Random Century, 1992.

Rayner, Claire, *The Body Book*, London, Piccolo, 1979.

Sayer, S., *Playing Safe: The Parents' Guide to Children's Safety in and out of the Home*, London, Thorsons, 1989.

Stockley, David, *Drug Warning*, London, Optima, 1992.

Thomson, Ruth, *Have You Started Yet?* London, Pan Books, 1987.

Wertheimer, Alison, *A Special Scar: The Experiences of People Bereaved by Suicide*, London, Routledge, 1991.

The video of *Safe and Sound* will be available in early 1993 from all good video stores.

INDEX